Table of contents

In times like these, we are all forced to change our usual routines and make adjustments. This currently affects almost all areas of our lives. It also affects any sports activity in a club or studio that is practiced in company, especially.
However, since it is essential for the health of the human body to exercise regularly, it should not be put aside – even in times like these.
I even think that in times like these, a correctly dosed exercise is even more important due to the fact that it strengthens our immune system.
Thankfully, there are many ways to exercise effectively from home or anywhere else without the use of equipment or with the help of very small devices such as the mini-band.
In the end, it does not depend on the provided conditions to move and do something for your body. It is up to every individual to start exercising. In this book I would like to give you valuable tips and accompany you on your way to a healthier and fitter body.
I have written this guide to help people to do their training easily and effectively from anywhere.

Introduction

We all do not move and exercise enough. The average European spends most of the day sitting. This is associated with many physical complaints and diseases of civilization; however, this need not be.

Overall, people today move much less than in the past. Only 45% reach the WHO recommendation of 150min exercise per week. And this rate is set rather low.

When asked why people do not move enough, there are usually many excuses.

Very often people are looking for problems and find excuses about things that don't fit. Consequently, people are annoyed. But this state only robs you of energy and does not get you any further.

Eventually, it is better to use the time given and deal with how to make the best of your current situation. Just like in current times like these. Movement needs neither much time nor expensive training equipment.

We live in a time with unprecedented possibilities – not just in sports, but in every regard. We have access to so many different things and maybe that is why we are overstrained and do not know where to start. When it comes to exercise, the decision should be quite simple. In sports it is not about what we do, but that we do something, it matters that we move.

Here are a few possibilities how you can do something effectively and reach your goals from any place by means of mini-bands.

But the first step to get started has to be taken by you!

This book is for ...

This book is for everyone who is looking for an effective training program that can be done at home, outdoors or any other place. It is also for those who cannot or do not want to go to a gym; and/or want to be flexible in their training.

It includes many different mini-band exercises ranging for beginners to advanced athletes. At the end of the book there are four different training programs. Additionally, the reader gets tips on how to achieve his or her goals.

Why you should train with a mini-band

The mini-band is a versatile training device that can be used to effectively train the whole body. An effective training can be achieved in a short time. Furthermore, the mini-band can be taken anywhere. Mini-bands are therefore ideal for on the go, because they fit into even the smallest pocket.

The many advantages of training with the mini-band

Because training with the mini-band is very effective and can be done anywhere, it is particularly suitable for exercises in the office, for travelers or people who have little time.

At the same time, it is a highly recommendable training tool for all people who prefer to train at home or outdoors rather than in a gym or for whatever reason cannot leave their home.

Hence, a diverse training is guaranteed!

Furthermore, the mini-band is very cheap and even if you buy them in a few different thicknesses, it will not put a strain on your wallet.

Mini-bands are used in every stages in training and sport – from beginner to advanced

A mini-band is a closed elastic band. It is another form of a rubber band, which is known to most people as Theraband (name of the market leader in rubber bands).

For years, these rubber bands or fitness bands were mainly used by physiotherapists for and in rehabilitation. Gradually, however, more and more coaches began to use them in training for their athletes. The ease of use and the effectiveness of training are especially appreciated with these elastic bands.

Today, the mini-bands can be found in sports and therapy equally and it can be said that they have made the breakthrough as a recognized training tool. And lastly, the mini-band is extremely popular with a wide range of people.

The colors of the mini-band indicate the level of resistance

The correct strength should be chosen with care. There are mini-bands available in different colors. The color indicates the strength and resistance of the band. The resistance is the decisive criterion for strength training. Hence, there is something suitable for everyone from beginners to competitive athletes.

It is recommended adding at least two different strengths for training. For example, for leg exercises you can usually use the stronger band and for arm and shoulder exercises the band with less resistance.

The most common colors and their resistors of mini-bands

- Yellow Mini-band – light
- Green Mini-band – medium
- Blue Mini-band – heavy
- Black Mini-band – heaviest resistance

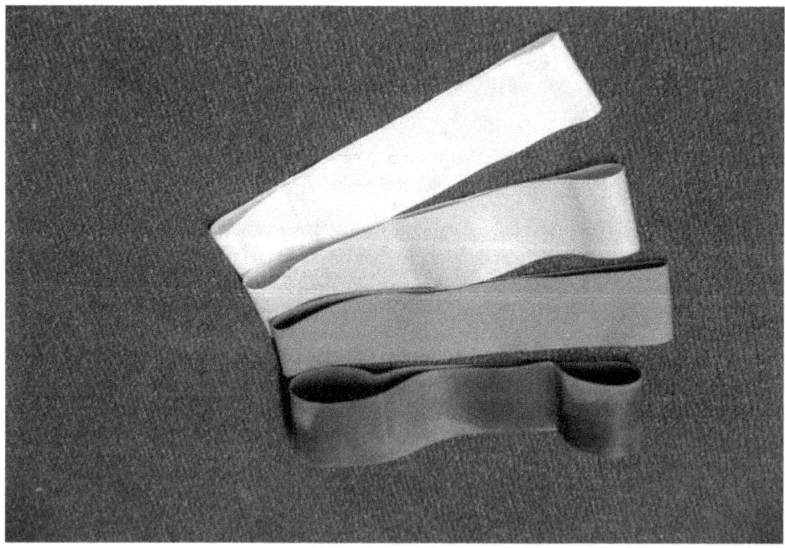

How to increase the longevity of your mini-band

Always use both hands to place the mini-band around your legs or feet. After the exercise, remove or wipe the mini-band again with both your hands. Do not shake off the band or step on the band with your shoes.

Additionally, avoid sand or stones getting on the mini-band. This can cause cracks.

Attention!
Mini-bands can tear and cause injuries if not handled properly. The tapes may be stretched by a maximum of 2 ½ times of its original span.

How to train with the mini-band

As with any other training, it is recommended to train regularly with the mini-band, preferably at least twice a week.

For starters – and/or if you have little time – I recommend you choose the best 4 exercises and repeat these 15-20 times per exercise. As an example, I have listed a quick beginner workout (for anytime and anywhere) below. You can then either do three sets of each exercise in a row or you can do the four different exercises in a row and then do three runs of them.

The training with the mini-band can be categorized as strength endurance training therefore you should take a break of about 48h between the units.

During this break you can still do sports. However, it is recommended ensure a balance in your training, for instance, easy endurance sports (e.g. swimming, cycling, easy running).

During the exercise, i.e. when the mini-band is pulled apart or the muscles are tensed, you should exhale. At rest, inhale slowly and deeply.

Before every training session, you should warm up a little bit, even when training with the mini-band. I will explain the importance of it below.

Tips to a Proper Warm-up

Why you should warm up before any training session

Warming up properly before every sporting activity is vital. It gets your metabolism going, prepares your body physically and mentally for training, makes you more willing to perform and – most importantly – reduces the likelihood of injury. Warming up also makes training more fun!

Here is why warming up is vital:

Going into training or a sports competition without warming up, you will feel that you get going much later and your motivation will be lower. More importantly, if you do not warm up, you run the risk of hurting yourself during training. This should be avoided in any case.

What happens with/in your body when you are warming up?

The body core temperature increases to approx. 39 degrees Celsius, the breathing frequency and pulse rate increase. This leads to a faster blood circulation which supplies the working muscles with more oxygen and nutrients. The increased heart rate also means that metabolic waste products can be broken down more quickly. For joints, ligaments and tendons a good warm-up program is essential. The body increases its synovial fluid, which is the name of the joint fluid that acts like a balm on the joints and athletic loads. The synovial fluid has therefore a cushioning effect on the body. By increasing the core body temperature, tendons and ligaments become also more elastic.

How you know that you are warmed up properly

The first beads of sweat appear on the forehead, your pulse increases and the muscles are in a pleasant state of tension, but at the same time they feel soft and supple. These are all signs that you are warmed up. Sometimes, this can be after 5-10 minutes. Sometimes it takes longer. This varies from person to person and always depends on what you are planning on doing. Generally speaking, the shorter, more intensive and faster the load is going to be, the longer and more thoroughly you should warm up.

If you plan on doing speed training, jumps or sprints, you should warm up much better than if you are doing a loose basic unit. If you are planning on doing a long loose unit on the bike, it is sufficient to start slowly with a low gear for the first few minutes.

As for training with the mini-band, it is sufficient to briefly activate the circulation, do a few jumping jacks and stretching exercises.

What can a warm-up session look like?

In general, a warm-up program should always be adapted to the kind of training or sport.

Depending on how or what you intend to train, your warm-up session should look differently. A warm-up always begins with a general warming up and activation of the metabolism. This increases the pulse rate and the muscles are warmed up and better supplied with blood. Further, more synovial fluid is produced in the joints. Afterwards, it is best to do some mobility exercises that you adapt to the activity ahead. If an intense shoulder training is pending or you are having a tennis match, your warm-up session will of course look different than when you go cycling. In order to increase the body core temperature and improve mobility at the same time, I will show you my favorite warm-up exercises in the chapter below:

Examples for a proper warm-up

If you are planning on training with the mini-band, then it is sufficient to do a brief warm-up. Ideally, your warm-up session should consist of two parts.

1. A holistic warm-up and activation of the cardiovascular system.

2. A precise warm-up and mobility exercises.

1. A Holistic Warm-Up and Activation of the Cardiovascular System

For example: jumping jacks, running in place, cycling on the ergometer, skipping/jump rope training, etc.

2. A Precise Warm-Up and Mobility Exercises (Mobility and Movement Prep)

Below you will find some exercises that will prepare you for the training ahead, but also increase your mobility. It is best to choose a few and execute them before starting with your training session.

More exercises are available on my homepage:

https://www.philipp-troschl.at/2019/07/18/aufwaermen/

or in my E-book *Fit at Work.*

Mobility exercises

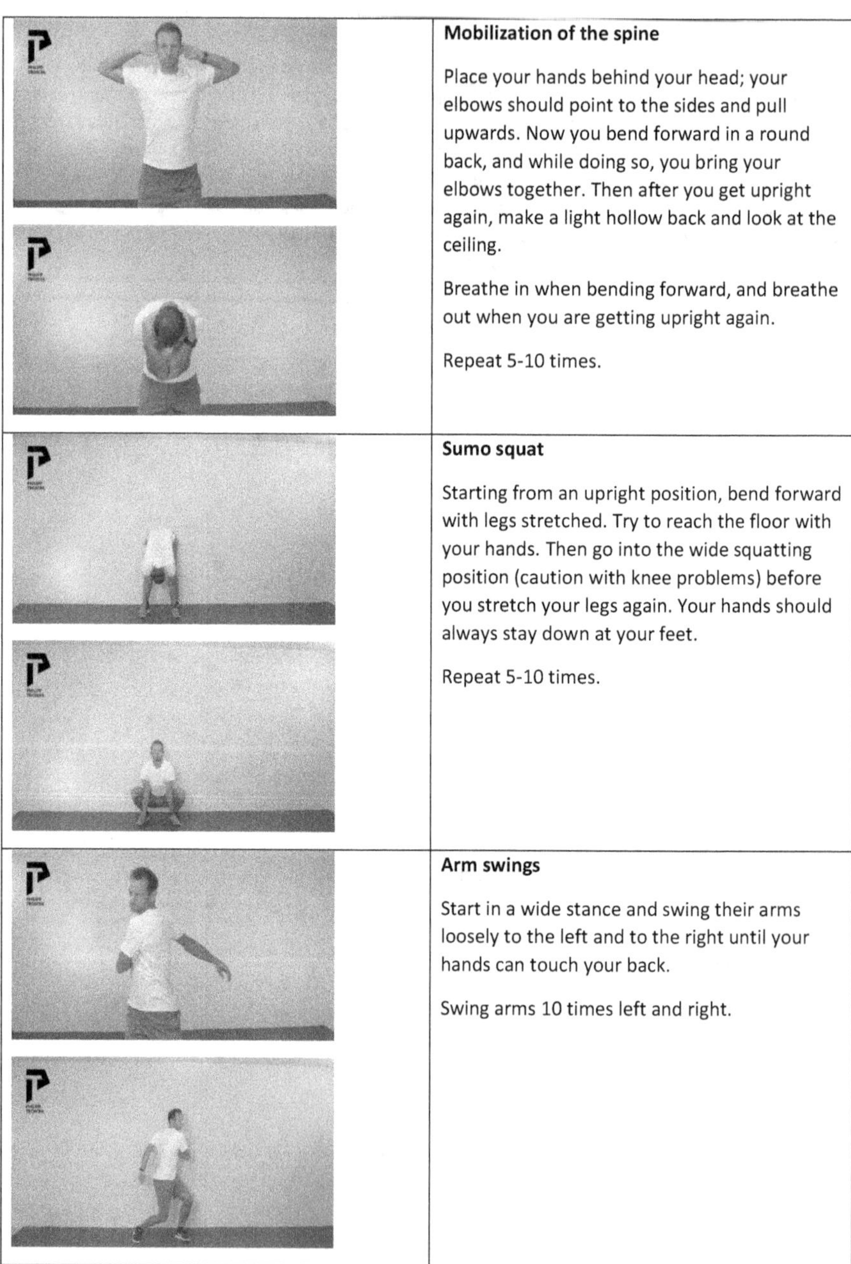

Mobilization of the spine

Place your hands behind your head; your elbows should point to the sides and pull upwards. Now you bend forward in a round back, and while doing so, you bring your elbows together. Then after you get upright again, make a light hollow back and look at the ceiling.

Breathe in when bending forward, and breathe out when you are getting upright again.

Repeat 5-10 times.

Sumo squat

Starting from an upright position, bend forward with legs stretched. Try to reach the floor with your hands. Then go into the wide squatting position (caution with knee problems) before you stretch your legs again. Your hands should always stay down at your feet.

Repeat 5-10 times.

Arm swings

Start in a wide stance and swing their arms loosely to the left and to the right until your hands can touch your back.

Swing arms 10 times left and right.

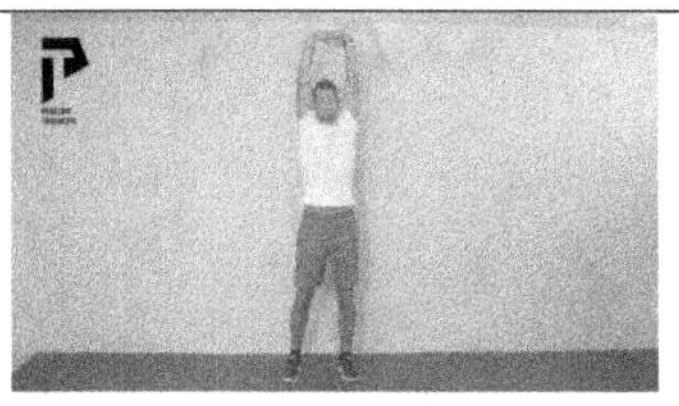
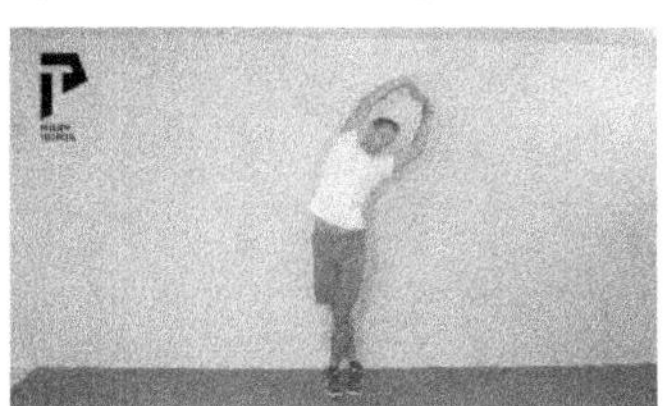

Side bend

Stretch arms upwards. Put your hands together; palms facing the ceiling. Place your right leg behind your left and now bend to your left. Stay in this position for 10-20 seconds. Then change position: put your left leg behind your right and bend over to the right side.

1-2 times per side; hold each side for 10-15 seconds.

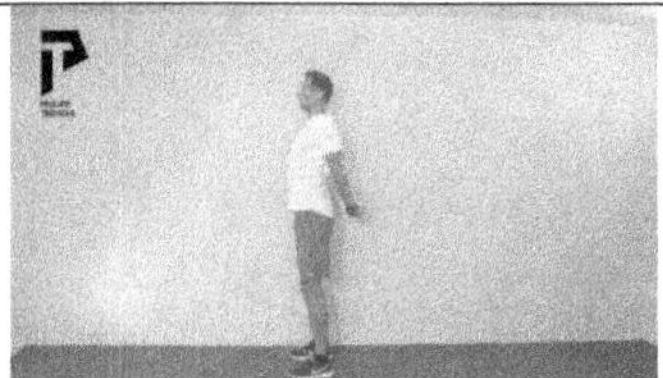
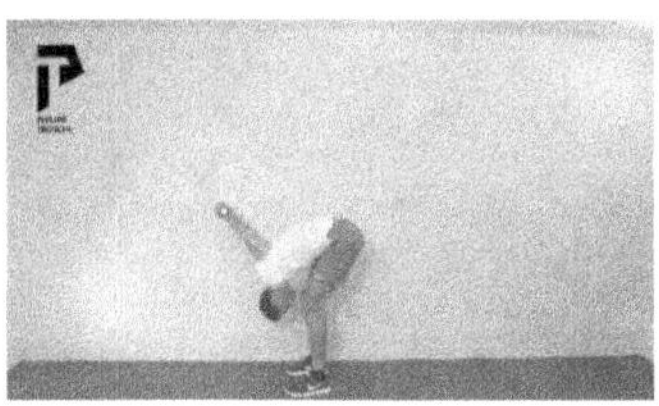

Forward bend with locked arms

Start in a standing position and put hands together behind your back. Now bend forward. First, do a hunchback (lower picture) and then look forward with your back straight.

If you have shoulder complaints please perform this exercise carefully. If it should hurt, then avoid this exercise.

Hold for 10-15 seconds.

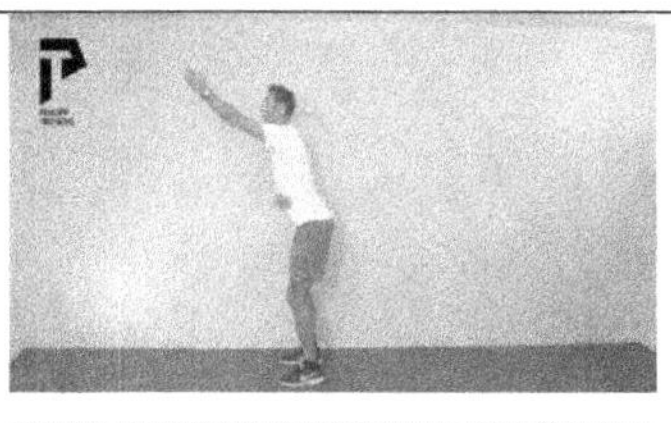
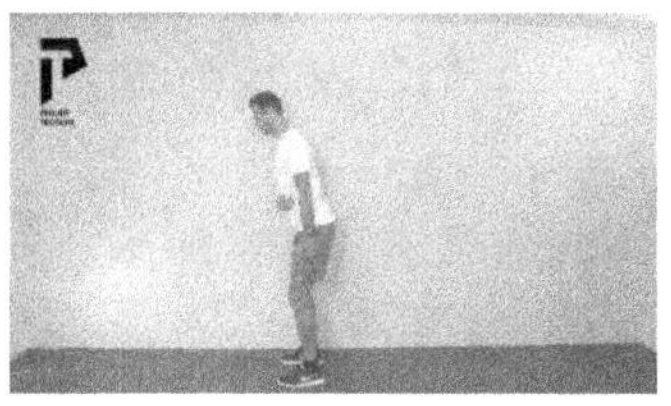

Arm circles

Place your right hand on your belly then draw circles with your left arm. Try to draw the circles as close as possible to your body. Now, switch arms.

Draw 5-10 circles per arm.

24 exercises with the mini-band for at home

Mini-band exercises in a standing position:

Monsterwalk (easy)

Lateral walk (easy)

Star excursion (advanced)

Lateral leg lifts (easy)

Squat (easy)

Squat + shoulder strength (advanced)

Lunge + shoulder strength (advanced)

Lunge and twist (difficult)

Knee lift (easy)

External shoulder rotation (advanced)

Mini-band exercises on the floor:

Leg stretch lying on the back (advanced)

Glute Bridge (easy)

Russian Twist (advanced)

Qaudruped arm pulls (easy)

Arm pulls in plank position (advanced)

Arm pulls in side plank position with bended knees (easy)

Arm pulls in side plank position (advanced)

Leg lifting in side plank position and arm pulls - Version A (difficult)

Leg lifting in side plank position and arm pulls - Version B (very difficult/pro)

Push-up and arm pull right/left (very difficult/pro)

Mountain climbers (advanced)

Mountain climbers with push ups (difficult)

Clamshell (easy)

Leg lifts sideways (difficult)

Monsterwalk (easy)

Starting position: You step into the mini-band with both feet and place it above the knees and thighs (alternatively also above the ankles on the lower legs). You start from a hip-wide stand, wide enough that the mini-band is slightly tensed. Then you go slightly into the knee and keep your upper body upright.

Exercise performance: You now take a big step forward with your right foot and then an even bigger step with your left foot. You can do this exercise in place or you can move forward or backward in monsterwalk. Make sure that you push your knees apart and that your upper body remains stable.

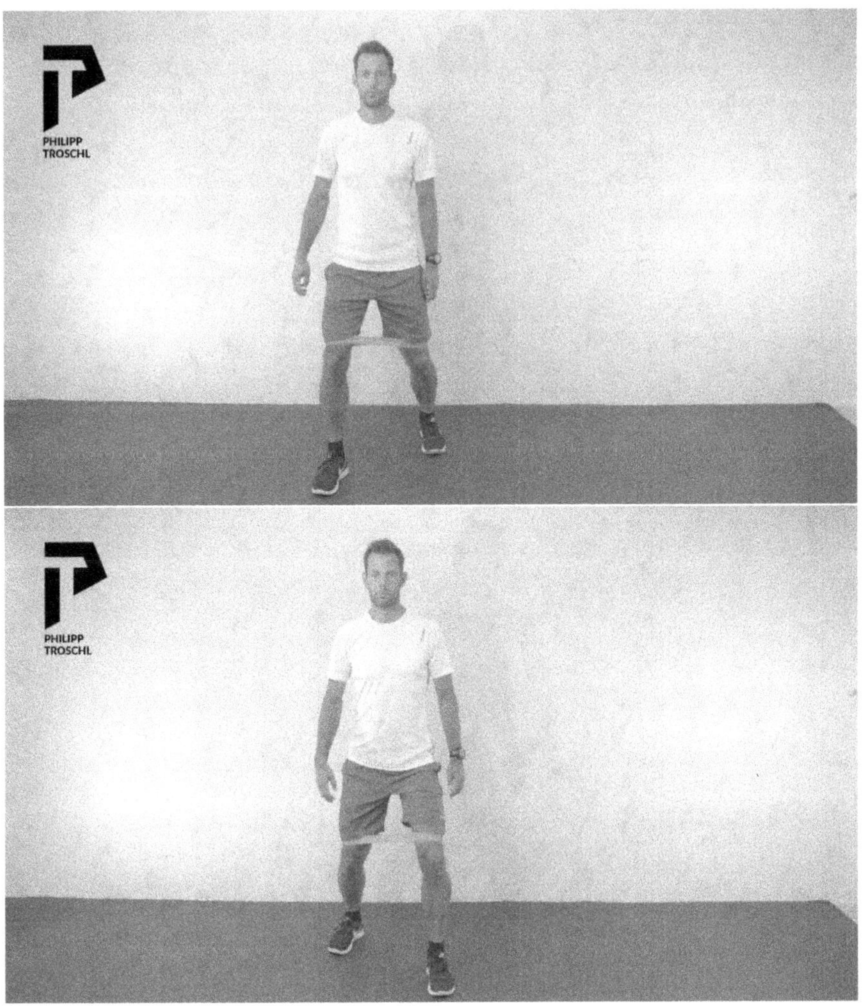

Lateral walk (easy)

Starting position: You step into the mini-band with both feet and place it above the knees and thighs (alternatively also above the ankles on the lower legs). You start from a hip-wide stand, wide enough that the mini-band is slightly tensed. Then you go slightly into the knee and keep your upper body upright.

Exercise performance: Take a big step with your left foot to the left side. Then make a small step with your right foot to the left, so that you can now make another big step with your left foot. Move like that for 10-15 meters to the left. Then do the exercise with the right foot.

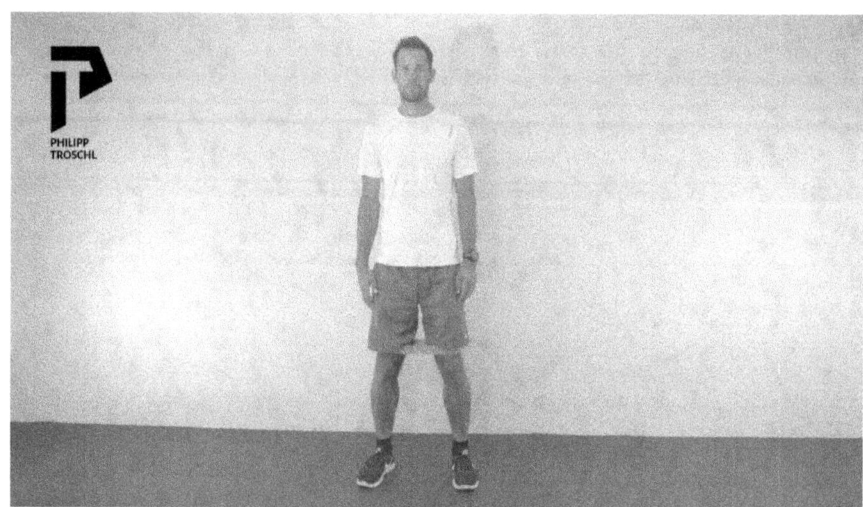

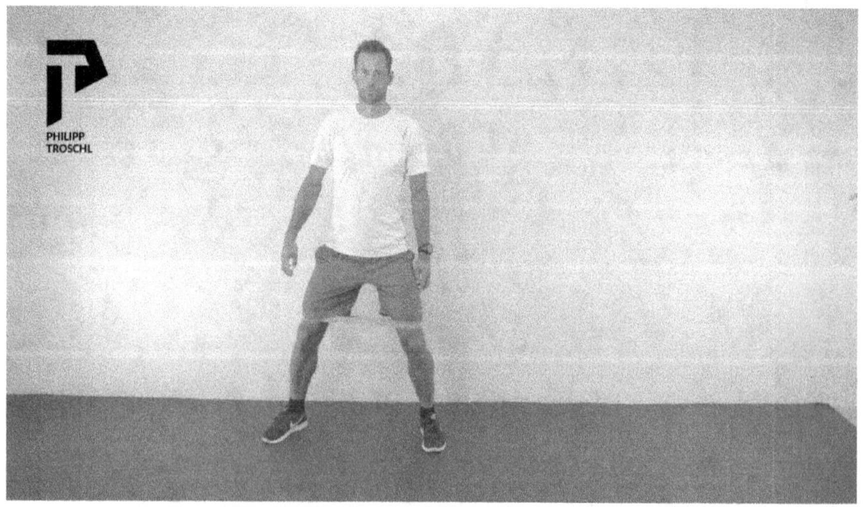

Star Excursion (advanced)

Starting position: You step into the mini-band with both feet and place it above the knees and thighs (alternatively also above the ankles on the lower legs). You start from a hip-wide stand, wide enough that the mini-band is slightly tensed. Then you go slightly into the knee and keep your upper body upright.

Exercise performance: Take a big step backwards with your right leg. Then back to the starting position. Then, with your right foot, step outer right and back again – and then forward and back again. Do this exercise **four times**, getting faster each time. Then do the same movement with the other leg.

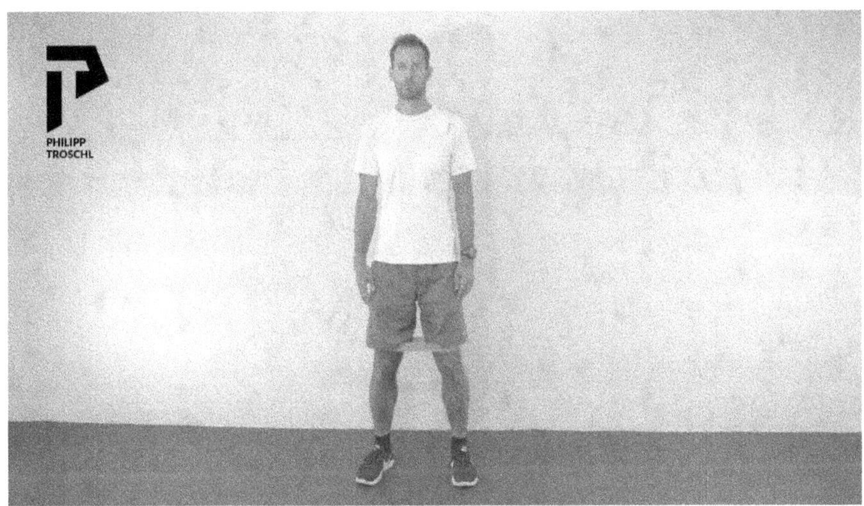

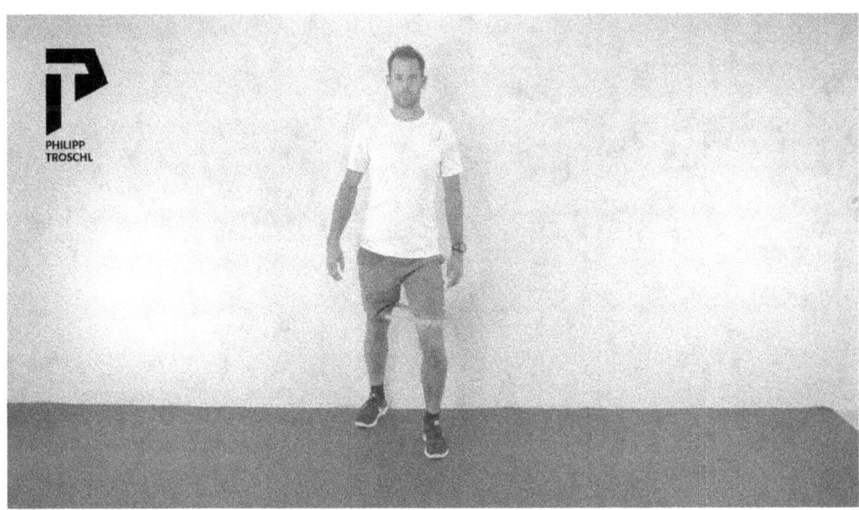

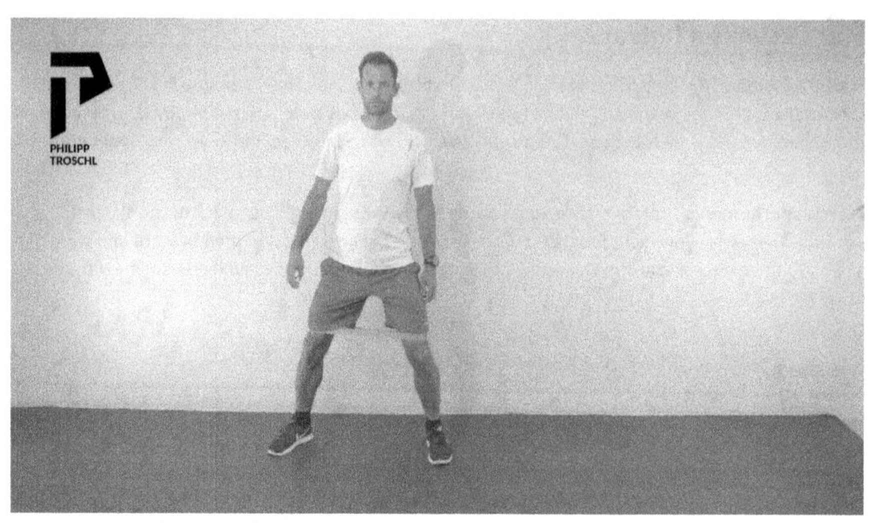

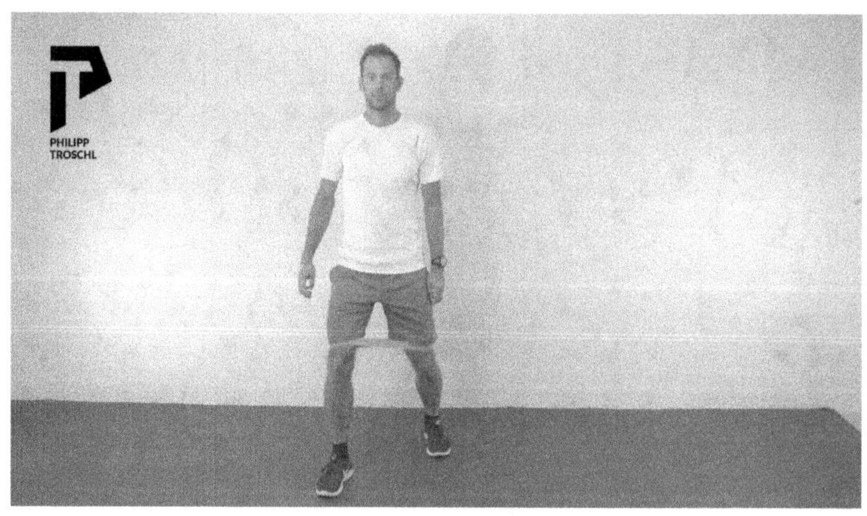

Lateral leg lifts – Strengthening of the Adductors (easy)

Starting position: You step into the mini-band with both feet and place it above the knees and thighs (alternatively also above the ankles on the lower legs). You start from a hip-wide stand, wide enough that the mini-band is slightly tensed. Then you go slightly into the knee and keep your upper body upright.

Exercise performance: You move the left leg outwards against the resistance of the band and slightly bring it back together again (repeat 10-15 times). Then you switch to the other leg.

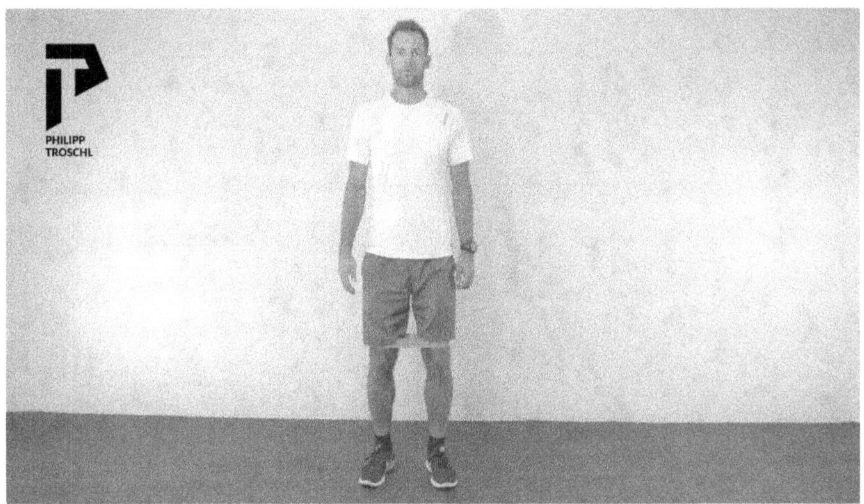

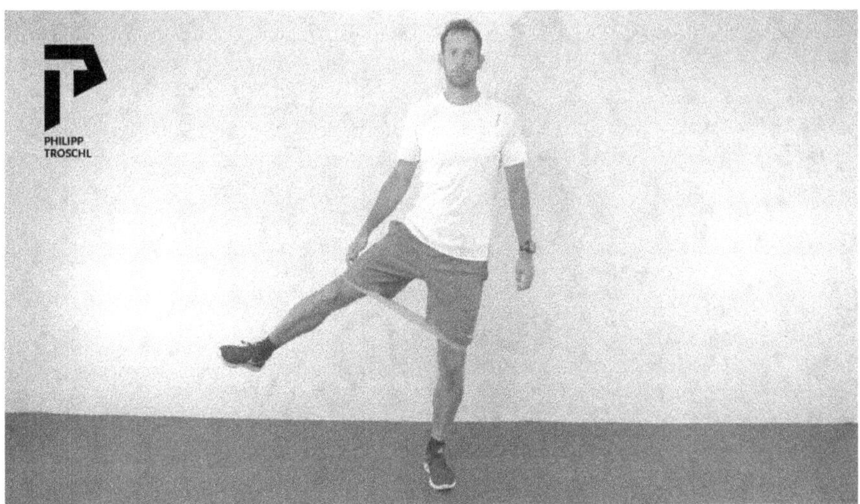

Squat (easy)

Starting position: You step into the mini-band with both feet and place it above the knees and thighs. You start from a hip-wide stand, wide enough that the mini-band is slightly tensed. Then you go slightly into the knee and keep your upper body upright.

Exercise performance: Push your pelvis back and bend your knees. As you move your buttocks back and downwards, shift your weight slightly backwards (on your heels). Now press your knees slightly outwards against the resistance of the mini-band. You want your thighs to be parallel to the ground. Your knees should not cross the front edge of your toes. Repeat 15-20 times.

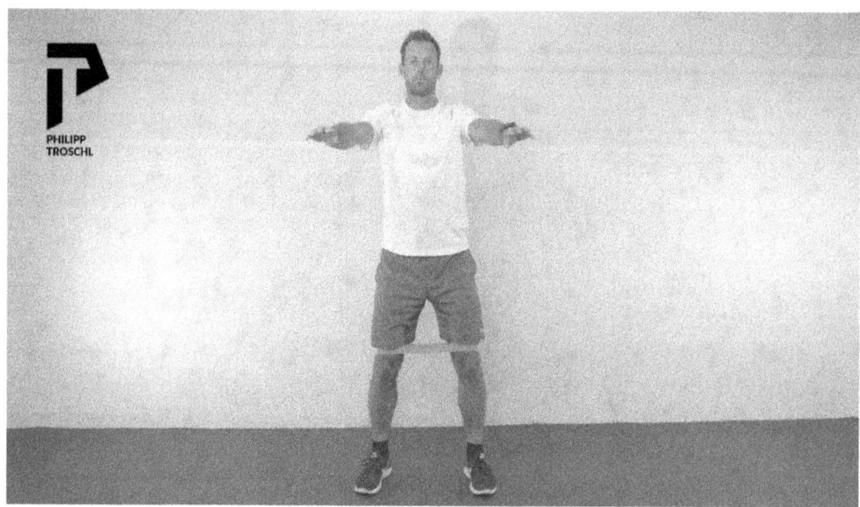

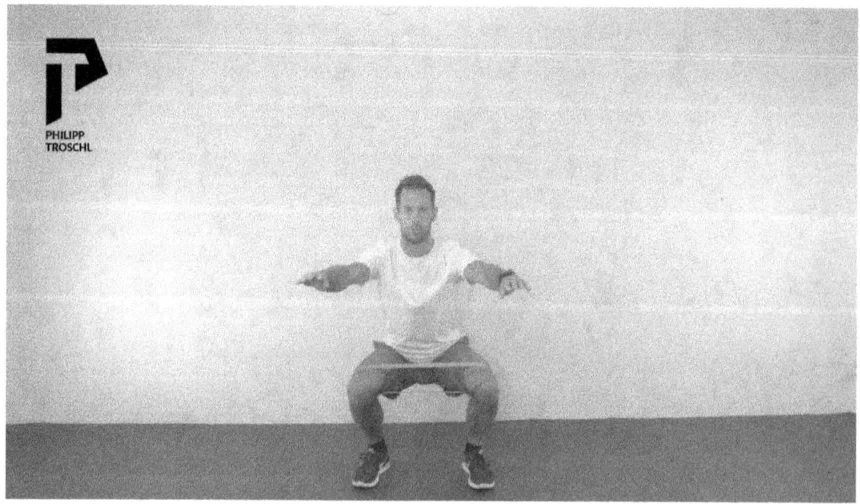

Squats and shoulder strengthening exercise (advanced)

Starting position: You step into the mini-band with both feet and place it above the knees and thighs. You start from a hip-wide stand, wide enough that the mini-band is slightly tensed. Then you go slightly into the knee and keep your upper body upright. In addition, place another mini-band around your hands and pull it slightly apart. Then squat and keep your upper body upright.

Exercise performance: Push your pelvis back and bend your knees. As you move your buttocks back and downwards, shift your weight slightly backwards (on your heels). Now press your knees slightly outwards against the resistance of the mini-band. You want your thighs to be parallel to the ground. Your knees should not cross the front edge of your toes. With your arms, keep the mini-band in a constant pull.

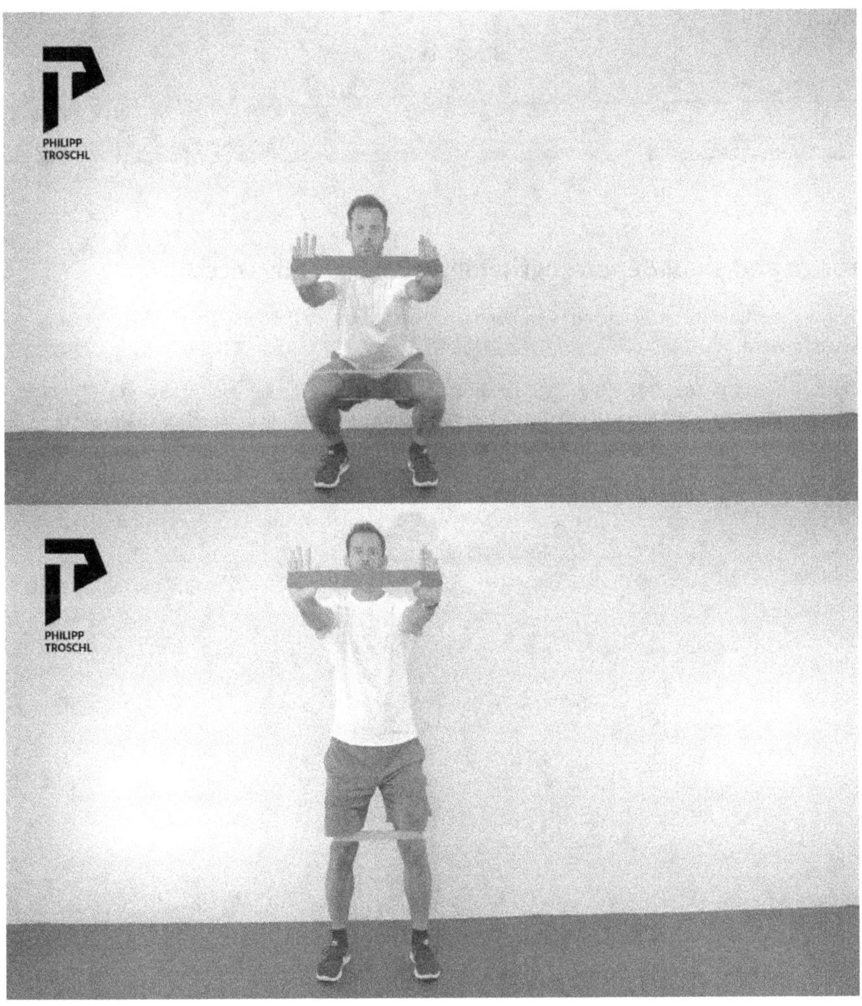

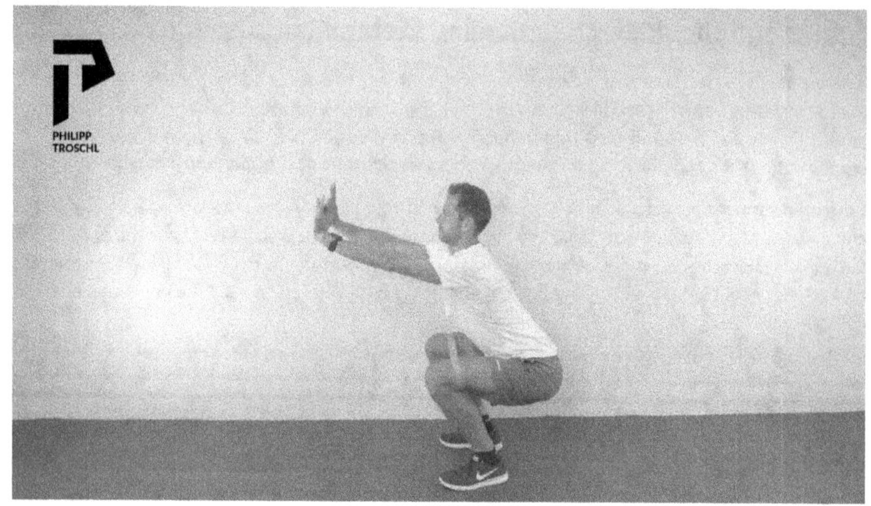

Lunge and shoulder strengthening exercise (advanced)

Starting position: Place the mini-band around your hands and pull it slightly apart. Now take a big lunge forward.

Exercise performance: Take a big lunge forward with your left leg. Lower your right leg to just before it touches the ground. Make sure that your front knee is approximately perpendicular above your front ankle when bent. Then stretch your front leg slightly to stand up again. Make 10-15 lunges per leg.

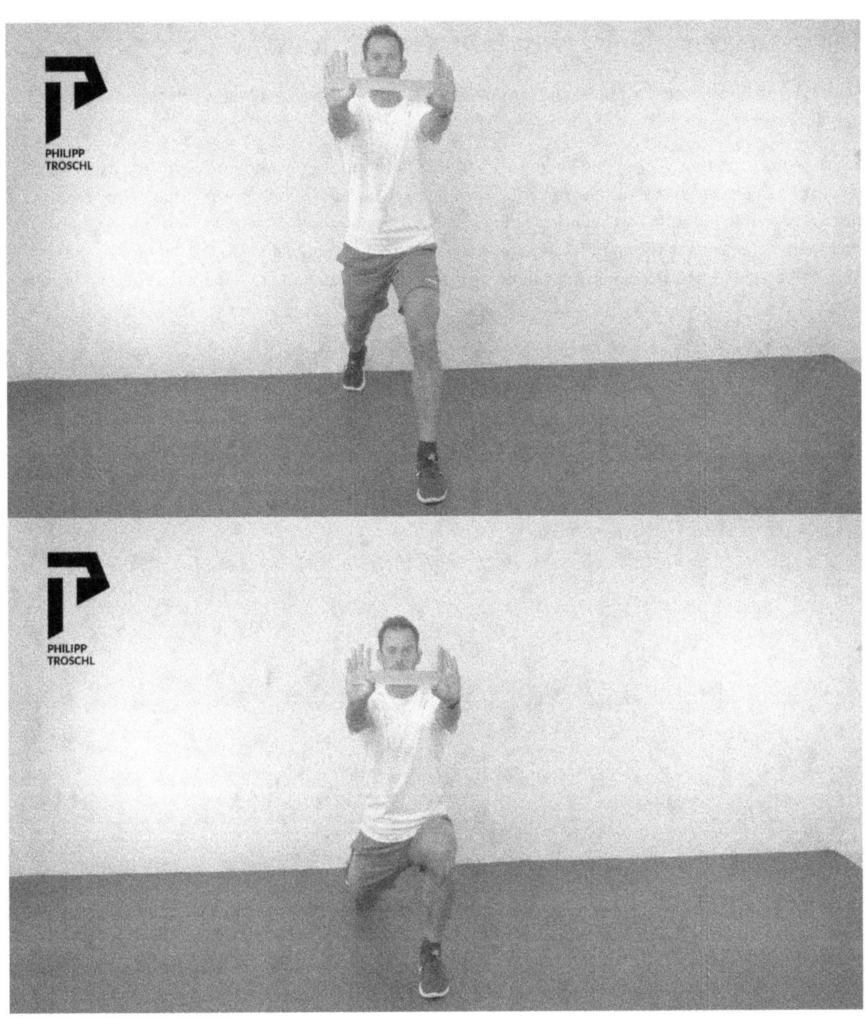

Lunge and upper body twist (pro level/difficult)

Starting position: Place the mini-band around your hands and pull it slightly apart. Now take a big lunge forward.

Exercise performance: Take a big lunge forward with your left leg. Lower your right leg to just before it touches the ground. Make sure that your front knee is approximately perpendicular above your front ankle when bent. In the lowest position turn your upper body 90 degrees to the left, back again and then 90 degrees to the right. Your gaze is always directed forward to the mini-band. Then stretch your front leg again to stand up. Then switch legs. Execute 10-15 lunges with an upper body twist.

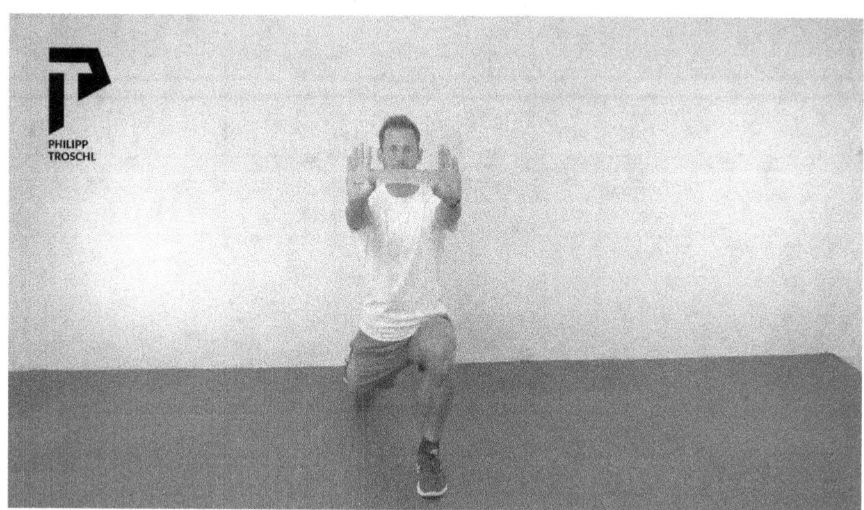

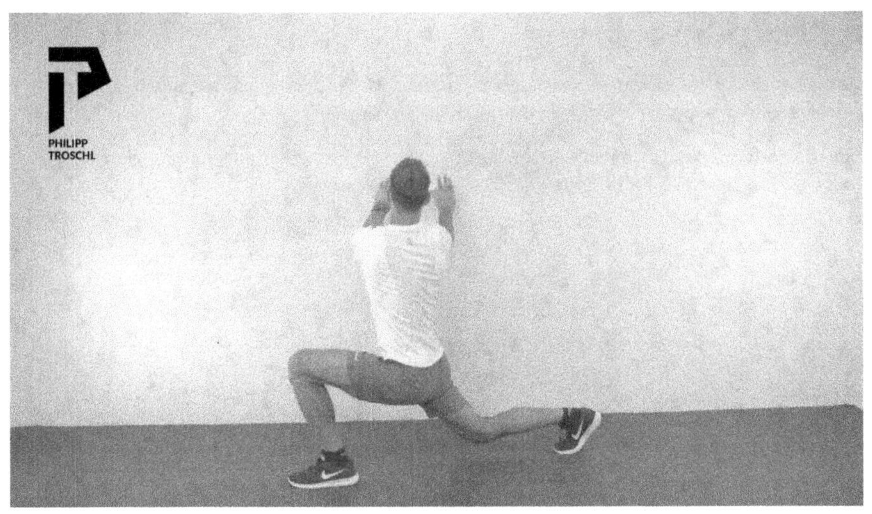

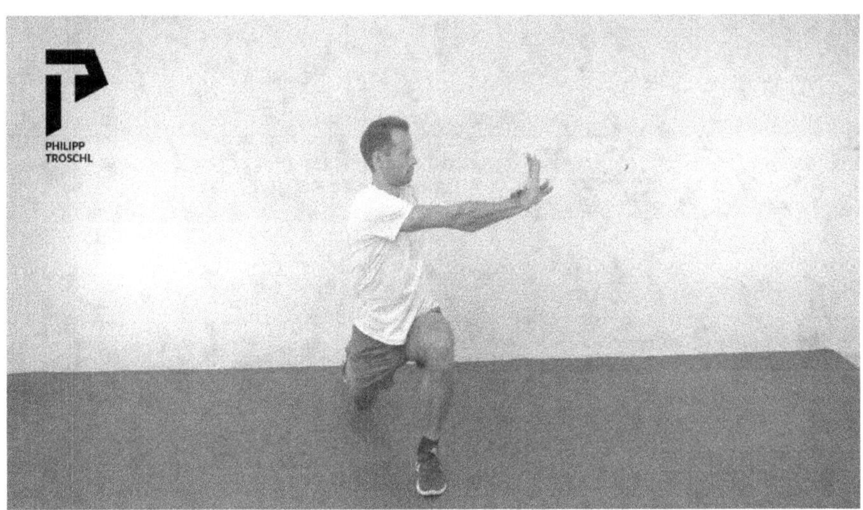

Leg lifting – hip flexor (easy)

Starting position: Place the mini-band around your feet. Make sure that you execute this exercise on a clean, rubber floor, otherwise the mini-band could get damaged.

Exercise performance: Lift legs alternately, against the resistance of the mini-band. Make sure that your upper leg is parallel to the floor.

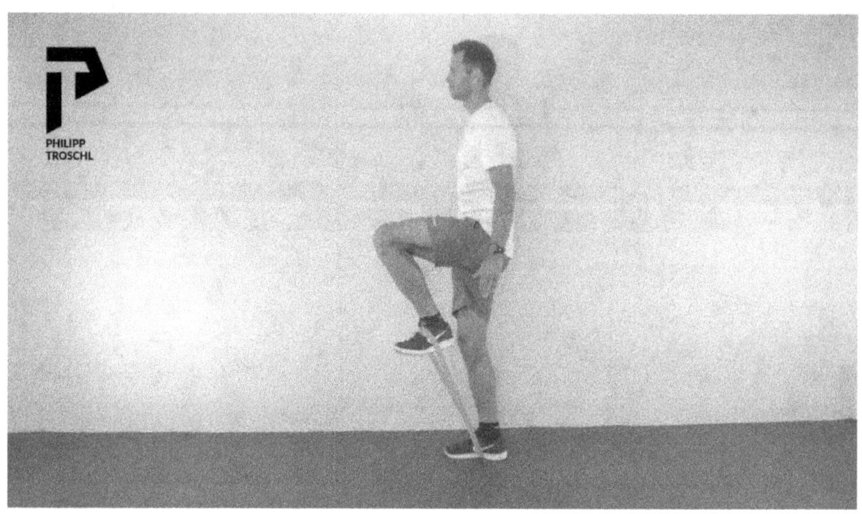

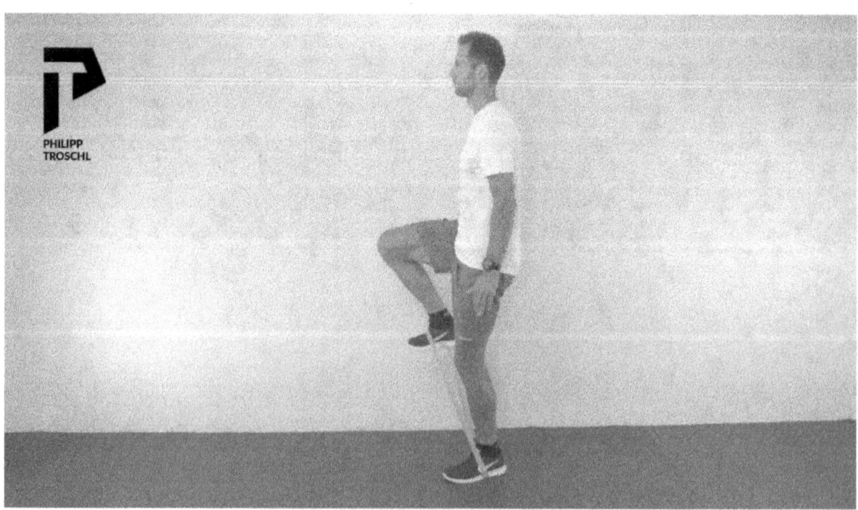

External rotation of the shoulders (medium/advanced)

Starting position: Put the mini-band around your hands (for this exercise a mini-band with a lower resistance level works just fine). Your elbows should touch your body and your shoulders should pull back.

Exercise performance: Now pull the mini-band outwards, making sure that the elbows stay on the body. When the mini-band is pulled apart, hold the tension for a short time before bringing it back together. Repeat 15-20 times.

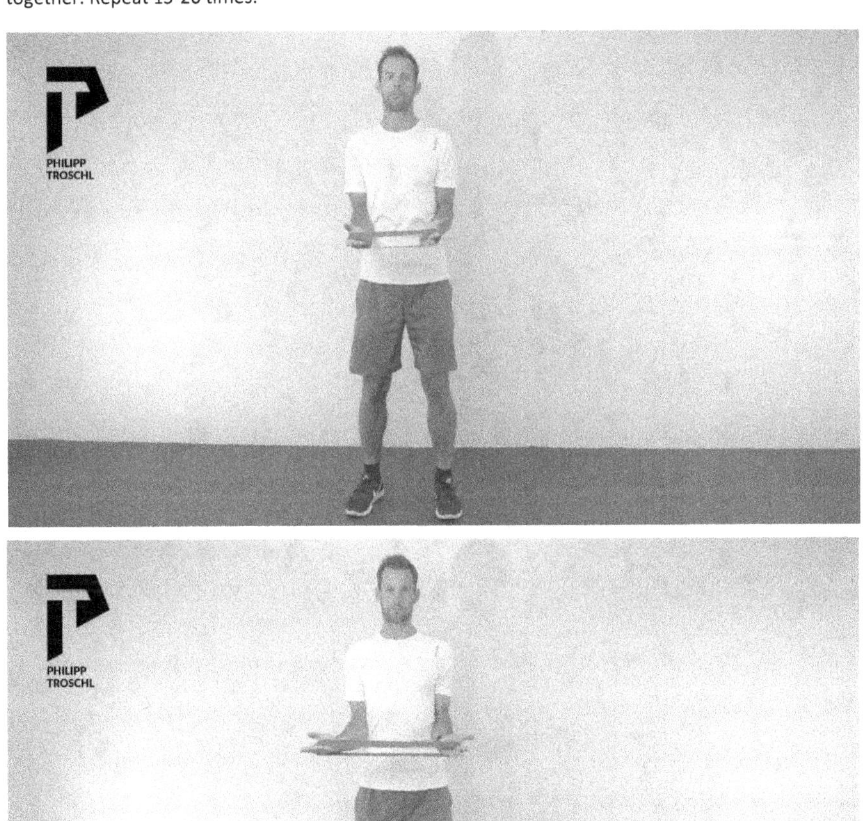

Leg stretching while lying down (medium/advanced)

Starting position: While sitting down, place the mini-band around your legs. Now lay down on your back and pull your legs toward your chest.

Exercise performance: Now, stretch legs alternately against the resistance of the mini-band. Hold the other leg in a stable position while the other one is stretched.

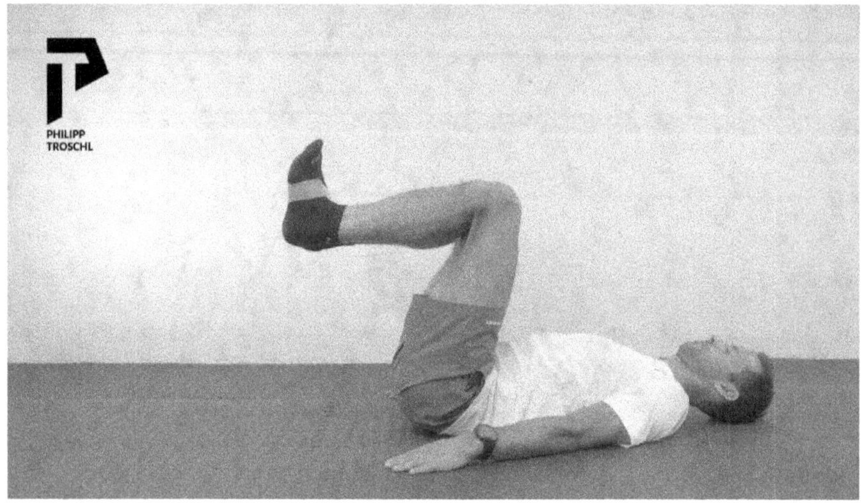

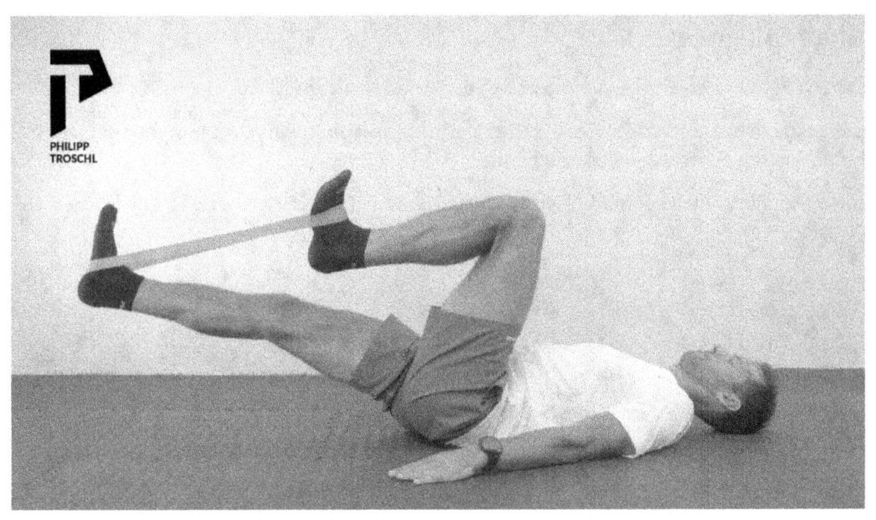

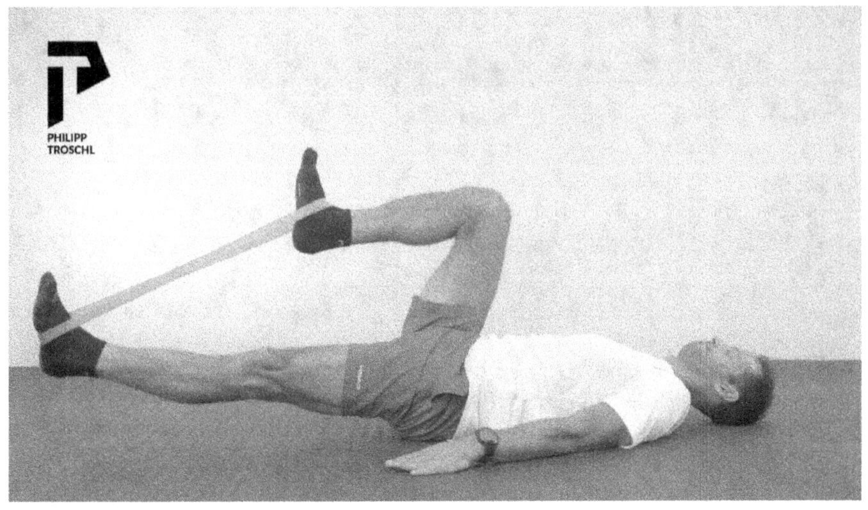

Glute Bridge (easy)

Starting position: Place the mini-band above your knees. Then lay down on your back.

Exercise performance: Now lift your bottom and make a full stretch in your pelvis. Hold this position for 1-3 seconds and tense your gluteal muscle.

Lower your bottom (do not touch the mat), before lifting and stretching your pelvis again. Repeat 15-20 times.

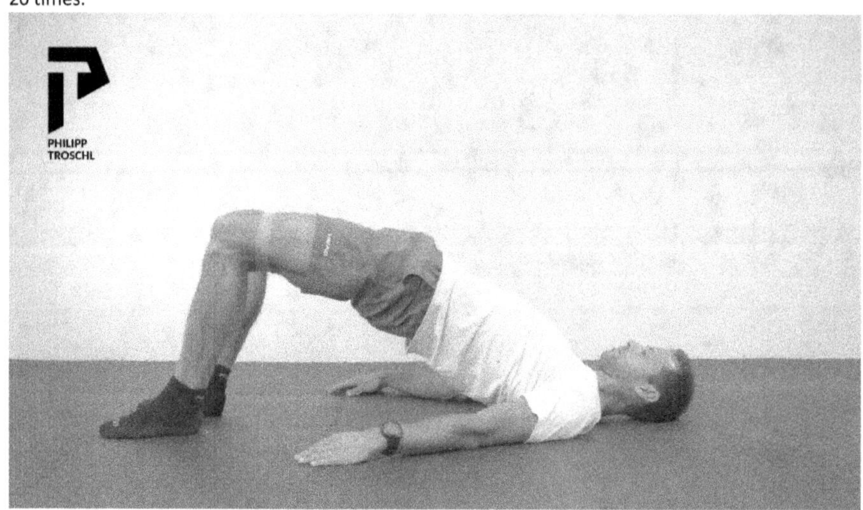

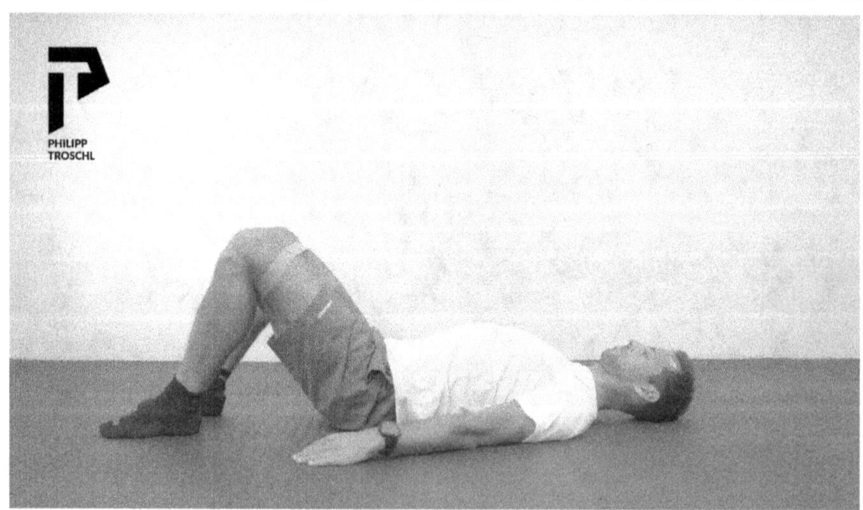

Russian Twist (medium/advanced)

Starting position: Sitting down, lift your legs from the floor and pull the mini-band outward with both your hands.

Exercise performance: From this position, turn your upper body and lead your stretched arms with slightly stretched mini-band once 90 degrees to the left and once 90 degrees to the right until just before the floor. Your eyes should always follow the movement of the mini-band. Repeat 15-20 times.

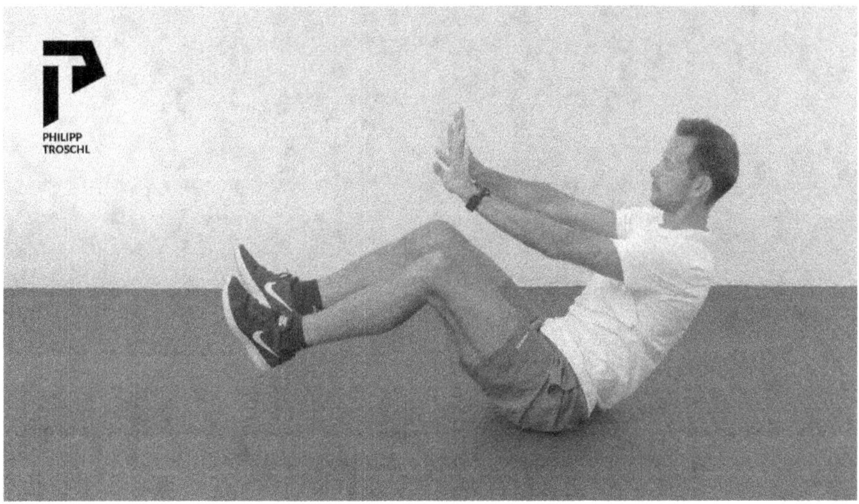

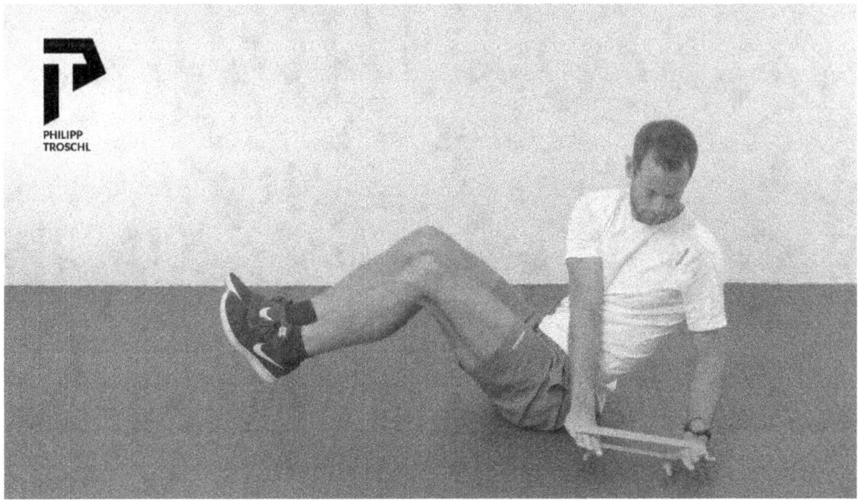

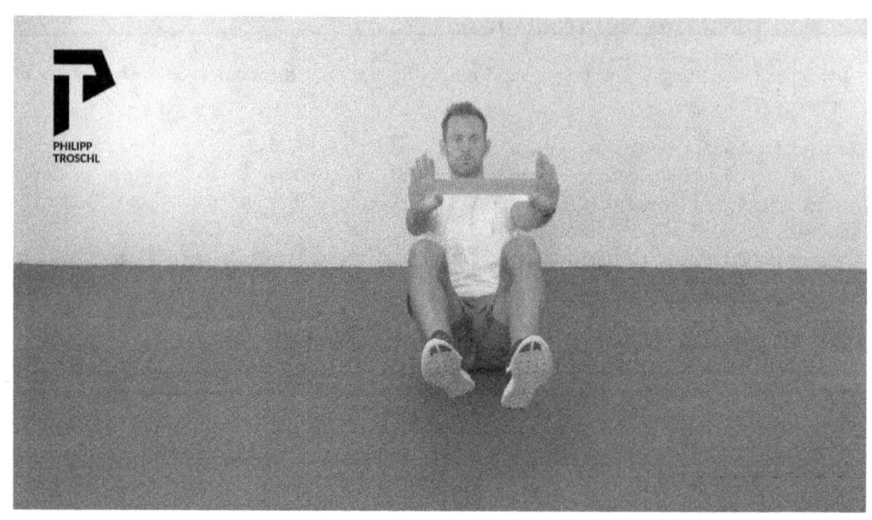

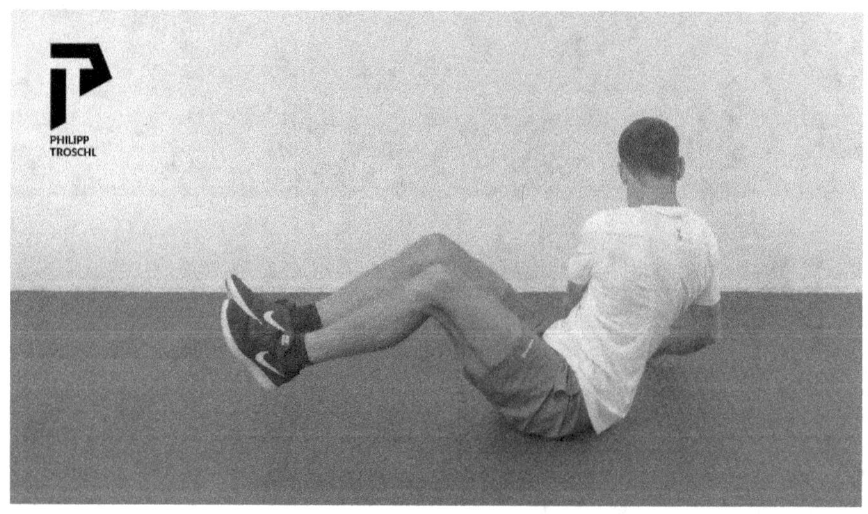

Quadruped arm pulls (easy)

Starting position: You start on all fours and put the mini-band around your hands.

Exercise performance: Now pull the mini-band with your left arm backwards and upwards. During this exercise, make sure that your elbow is pulled upwards just past your body. Then, switch arms. Repeat 15-20 times per arm.

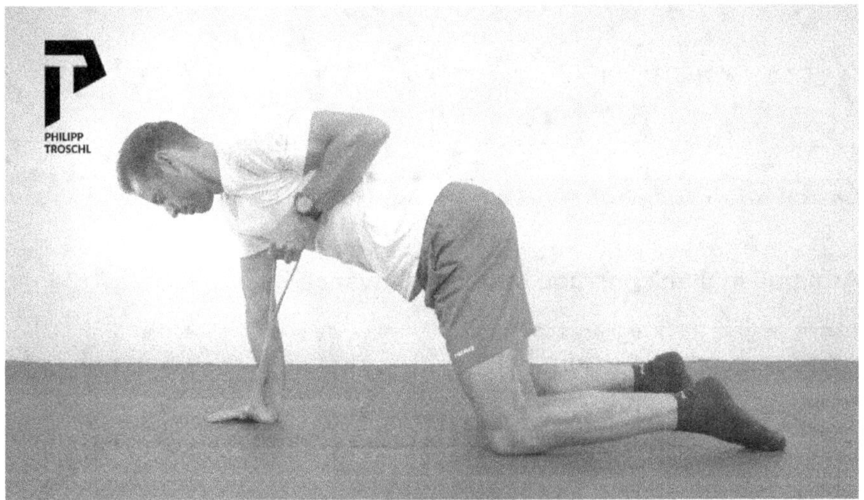

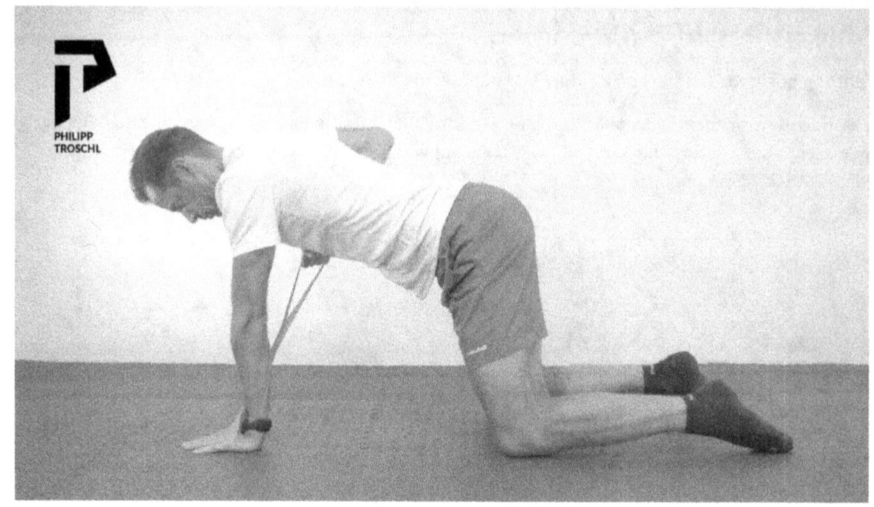

Arm pull in plank position (medium/advanced)

Starting position: Start in plank position and put the mini-band around your hands.

Exercise performance: Now pull the mini-band with your left arm backwards and upwards. During this exercise, make sure that your elbow is pulled upwards just past your body. Now switch arms. Repeat 15-20 times. Alternatively, you can alternate arms in between.

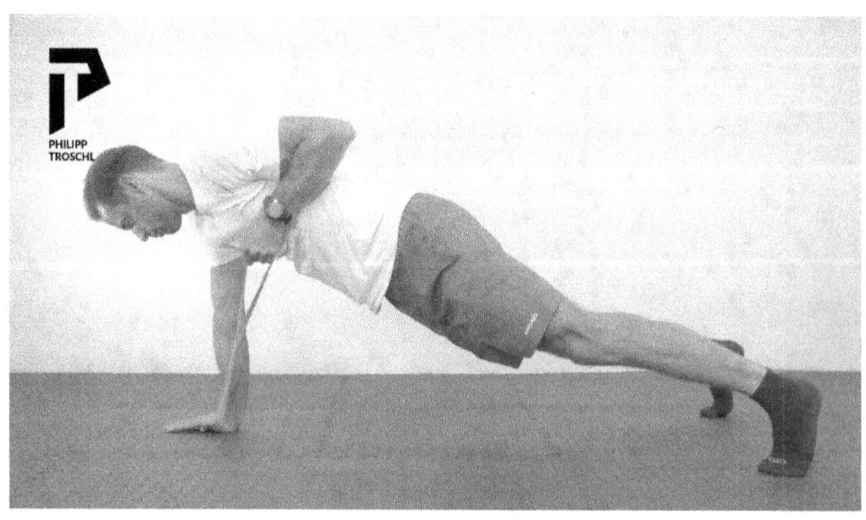

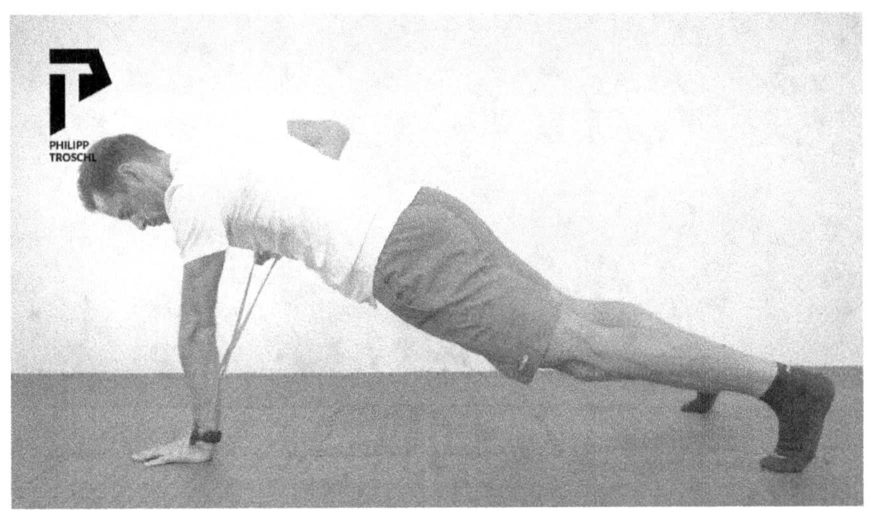

Arm pull in side plank position with knees bended 90 degree (easy)

Starting position: You start in a side plank position and bend your knees in a 90-degree angle. Your right elbow should be located vertically under your right shoulder. The thighs and upper body form a line and the hips are fully extended. Put the mini-band around your hands.

Exercise performance: Now pull the mini-band back and upwards with your left arm. Make sure that

your elbow is close to your body while pull in the band. Then, switch sides. Repeat 15-20 times per side.

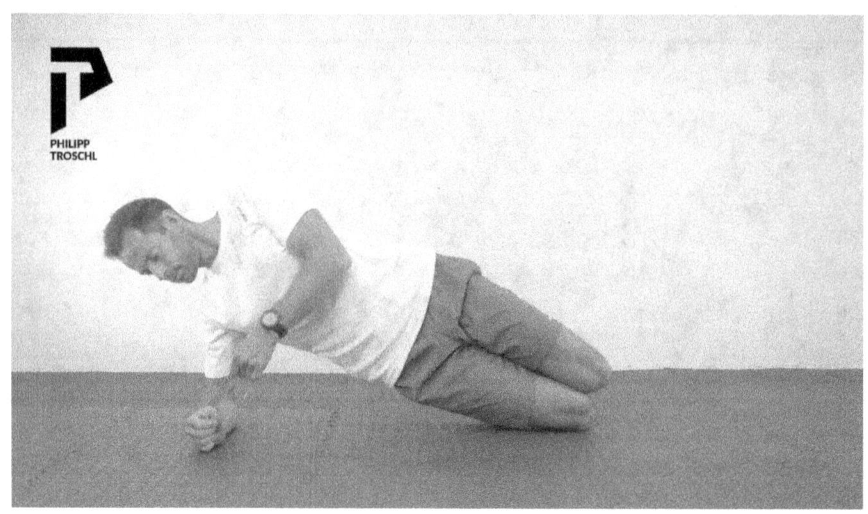

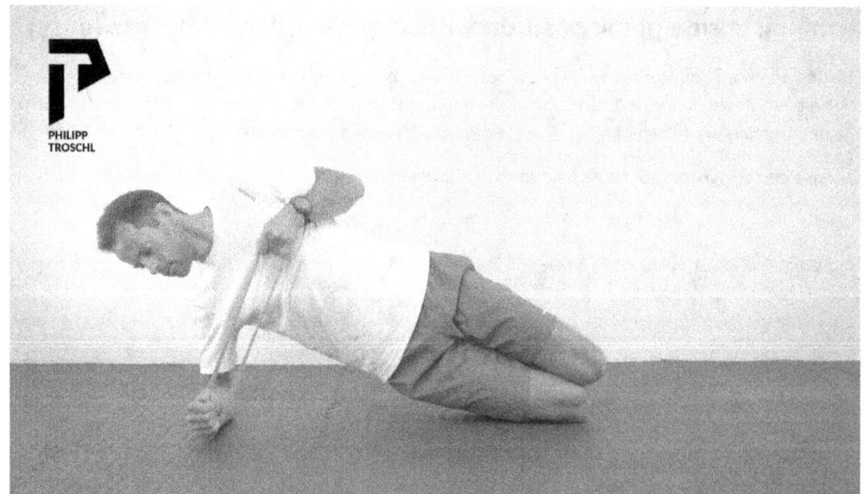

Arm pull in side plank position with stretched out legs (medium/advanced)

Starting position: You start in a side plank position and stretched out legs. Your right elbow should be located vertically under your right shoulder. The thighs and upper body form a line and the hips are fully extended. Put the mini-band around your hands.

Exercise performance: Now pull the mini-band back and upwards with your left arm. Make sure that your elbow is close to your body while pull in the band. Then, switch sides. Repeat 15-20 times per side.

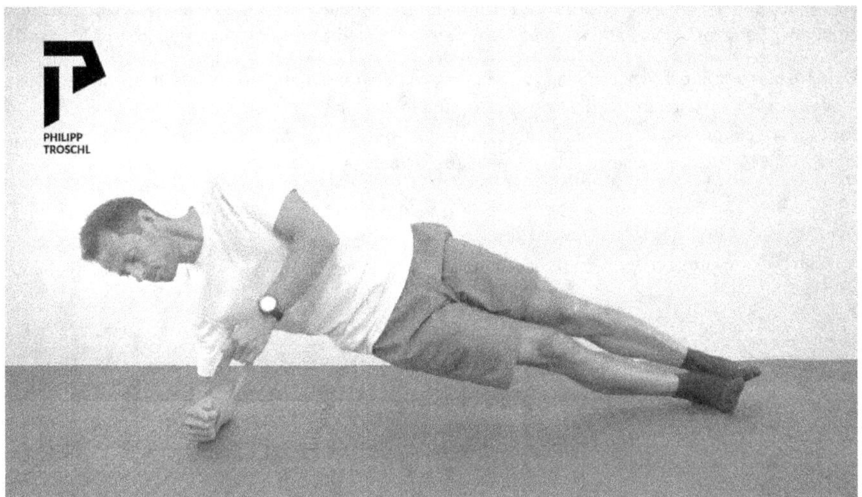

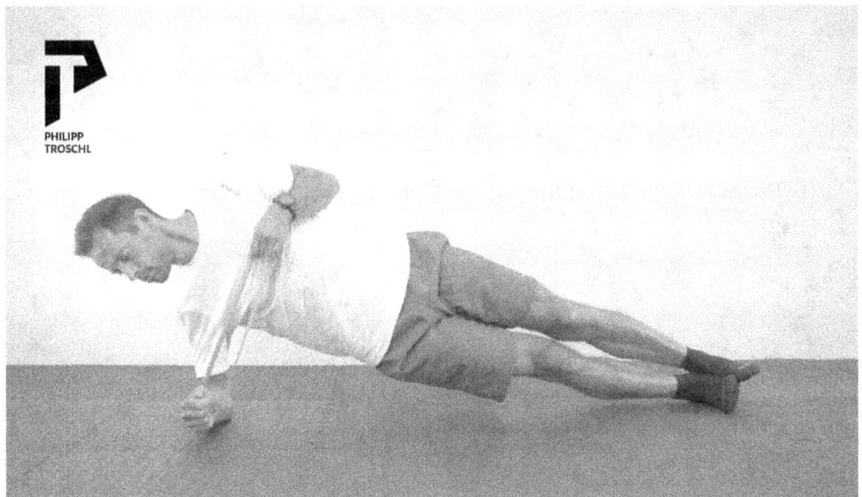

Leg lifting in side plank position and arm pulls - Version A (difficult)

Starting position: You start in side plank position and bend your knees in a 90-degree angle. Your right elbow should be located vertically under your right shoulder. Now lift the leg on top. The thighs and upper body form a line and the hips are fully extended. Put the mini-band around your hands.

Exercise performance: While pulling the mini-band with your left arm backwards and upwards you move your left leg outwards and upwards. Keep the tension in your torso area and make sure that the hips are completely stretched. During this exercise, make sure that your elbow is pulled upwards close to your body. Then change sides. Repeat 15-20 times per side.

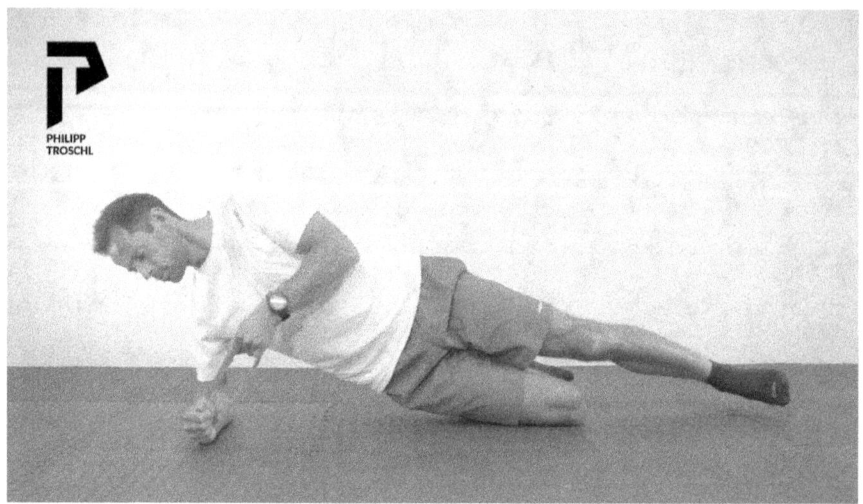

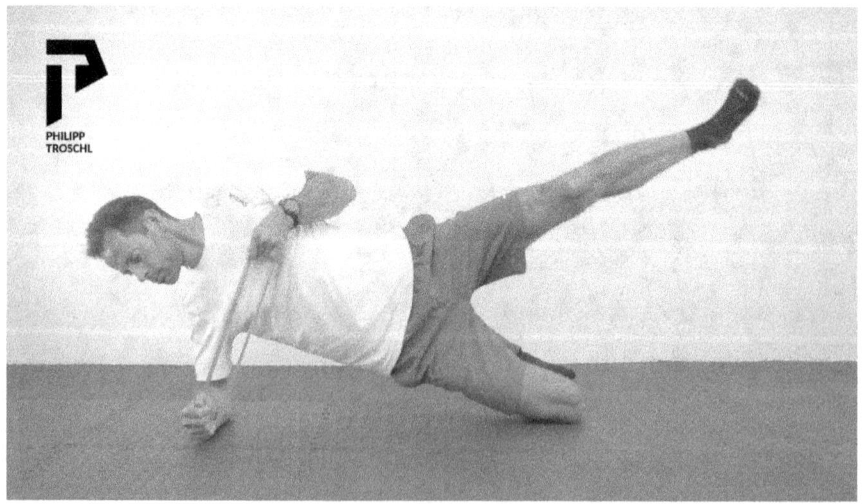

Leg lifting in side plank position and arm pulls Version B (very difficult/pro)

Starting position: You start in a side plank position and bend your knees in a 90-degree angle. Your right elbow should be located vertically under your right shoulder. Now lift the leg on top. The thighs and upper body form a line and the hips are fully extended. Put the mini-band around your hands.

Exercise performance: While pulling the mini-band with your left arm backwards and upwards you move your left leg outwards and upwards. Keep the tension in your torso area and make sure that the hips are completely stretched. During this exercise, make sure that your elbow is pulled upwards close to your body. Then change sides. Repeat 15-20 times per side.

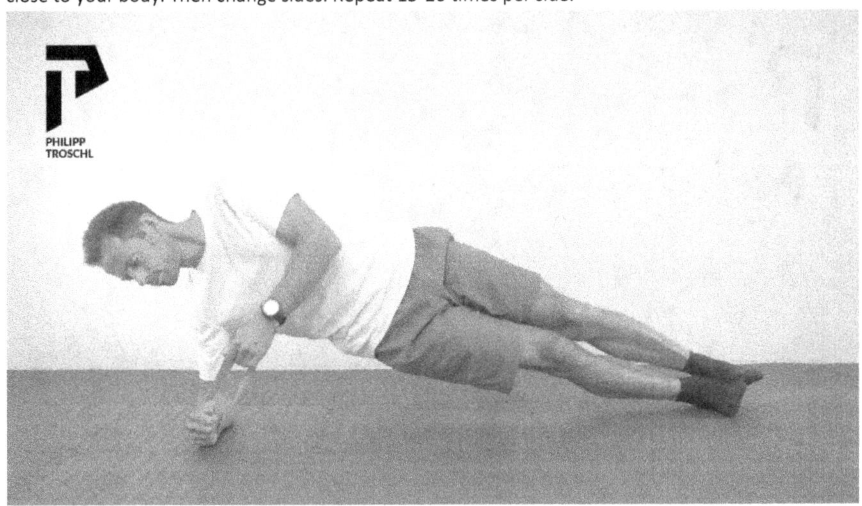

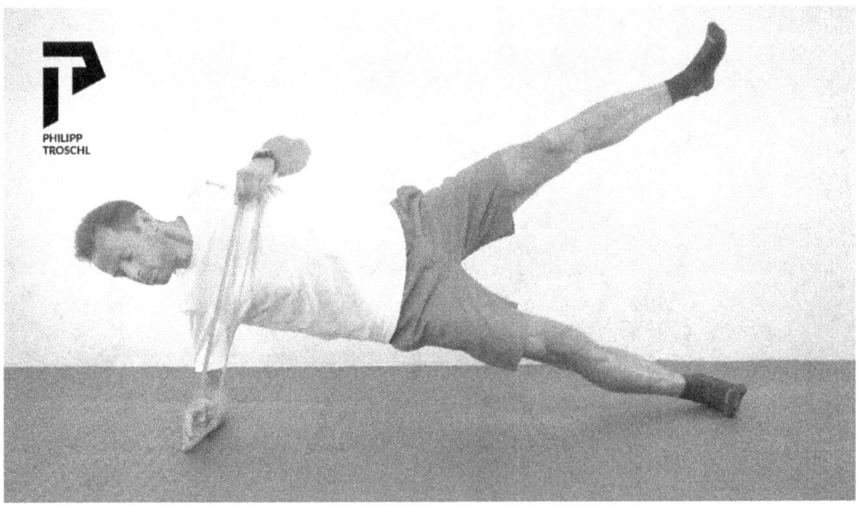

Push-up and arm pull right/left (very difficult/pro)

Starting position: You start this exercise in plank position and place the mini-band around your hands.

Exercise performance: While pulling the mini-band with your left arm backwards and upwards you move your left leg outwards and upwards. During this exercise, make sure that your elbow is pulled upwards close to your body. Do a push-up (again elbows should stay close to your body) and then pull the mini-band upwards with your right arm. Alternatively, you can opt for switching arms in-between the push-ups. Repeat 15-20 times.

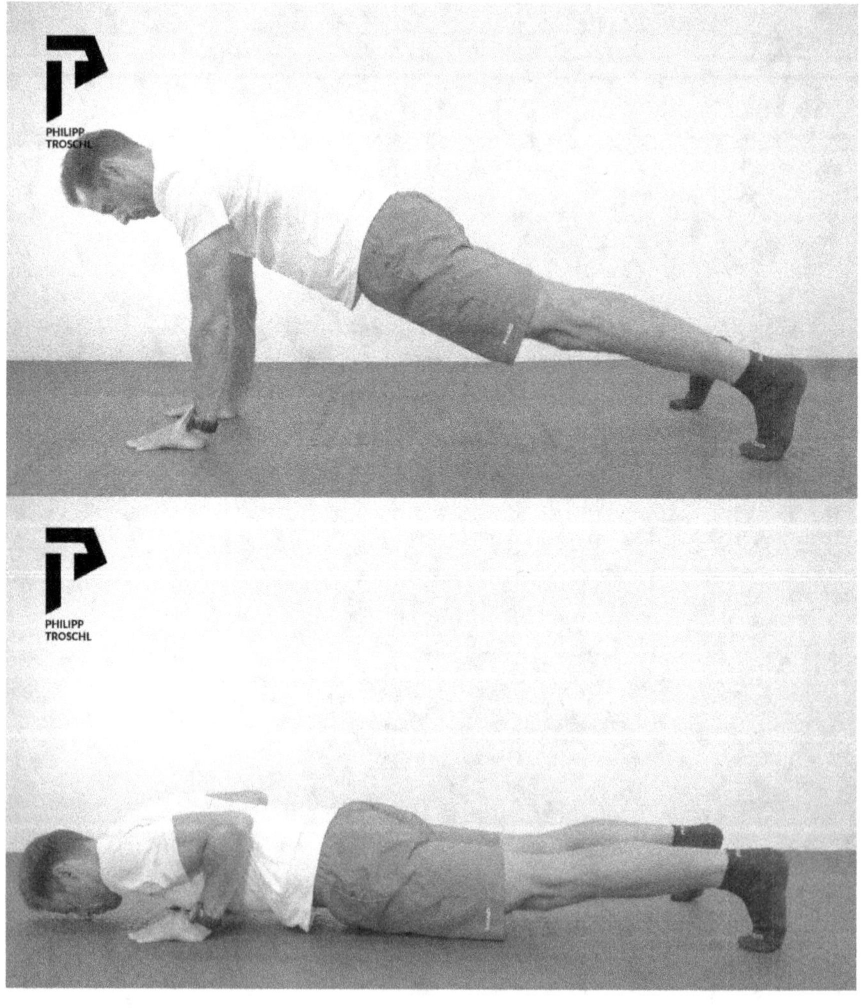

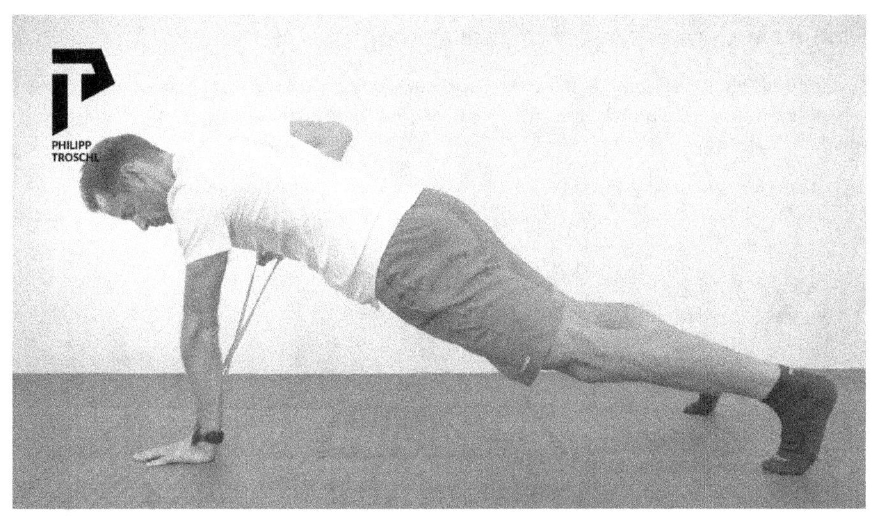

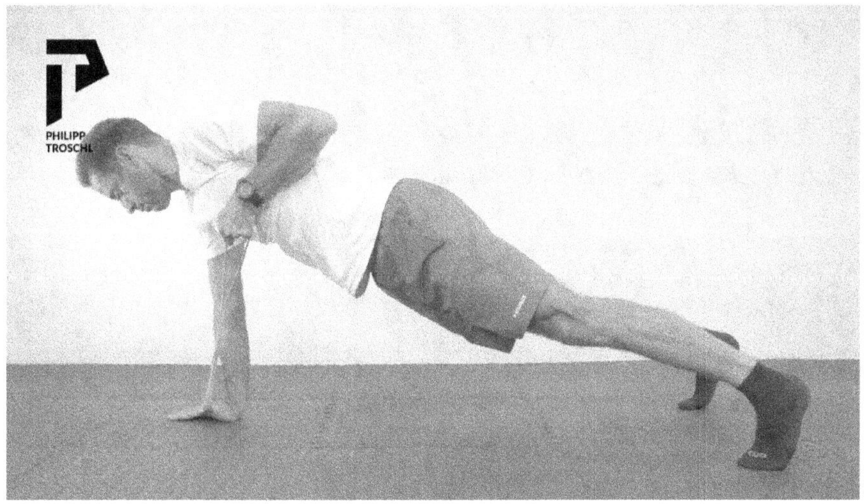

Mountain climbers (medium/advanced)

Starting position: You start this exercise in plank position and place a mini-band around your hands, as well as one around your feet. Stretch the mini-band with your hands slightly, but just enough so you can fell a resistance.

Exercise performance: Now you pull the mini-band with your right foot by making a big step forward. Step back and switch legs. You can also try alternating jumps. Repeat 10-20 times.

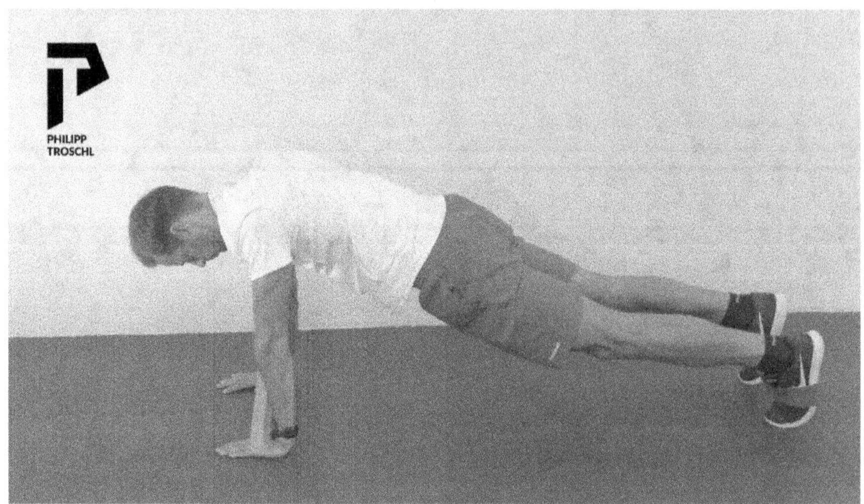

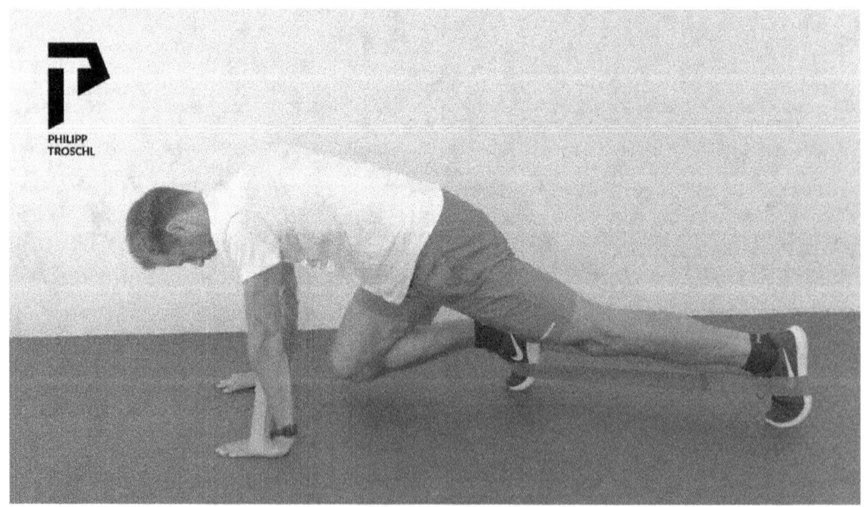

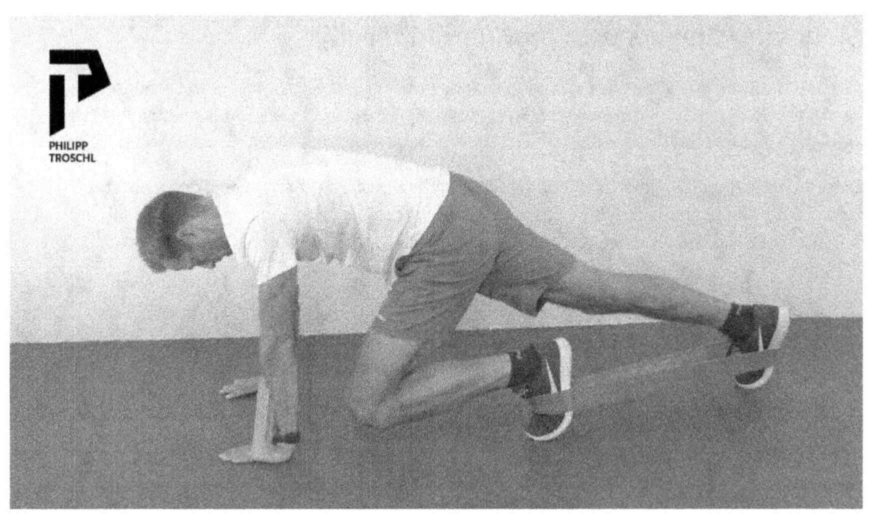

PHILIPP
TROSCHL

Mountain climbers with push-ups (difficult)

Starting position: You start this exercise in a plank position and place a mini-band around your hands, as well as one around your feet. Stretch the mini-band with your hands slightly, but just enough so you can fell a resistance.

Exercise performance: Now you pull the mini-band with your right foot by making a big step forward. Step back and switch legs. You can also try alternating jumps. After every step left and right, you make one push-up. Repeat 10-20 times.

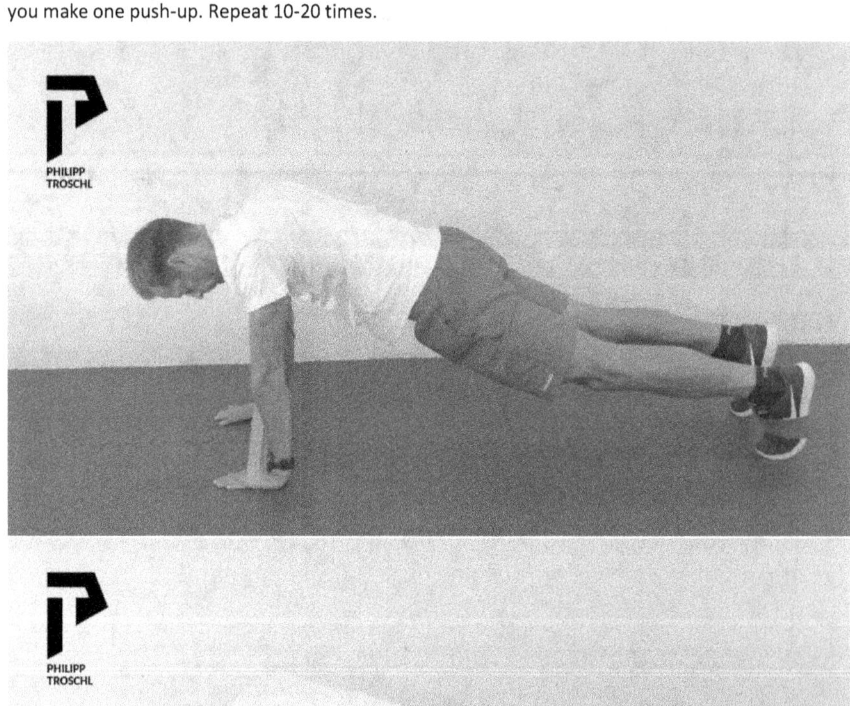

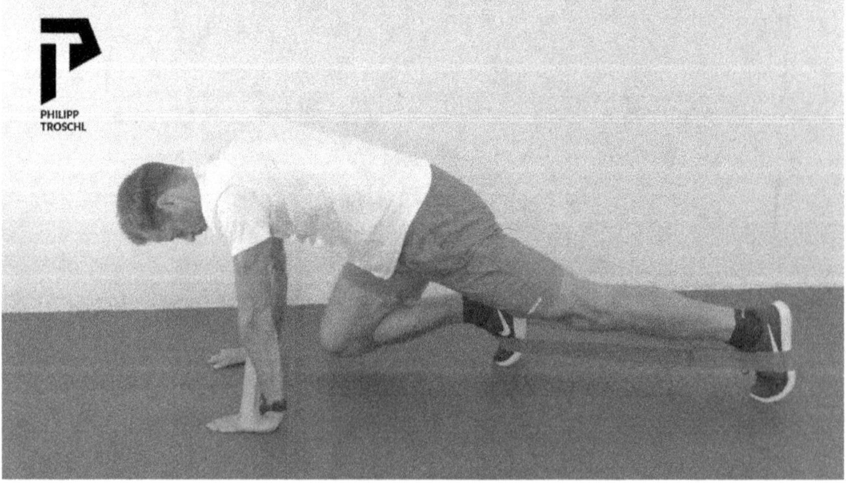

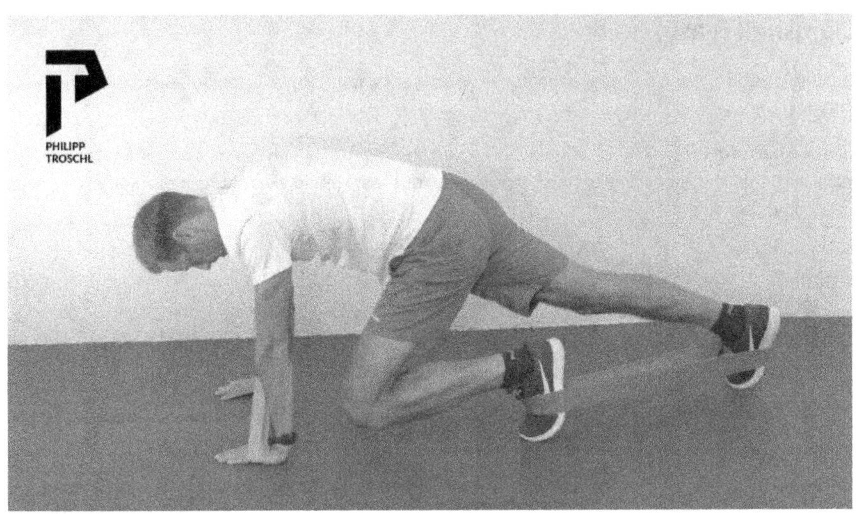

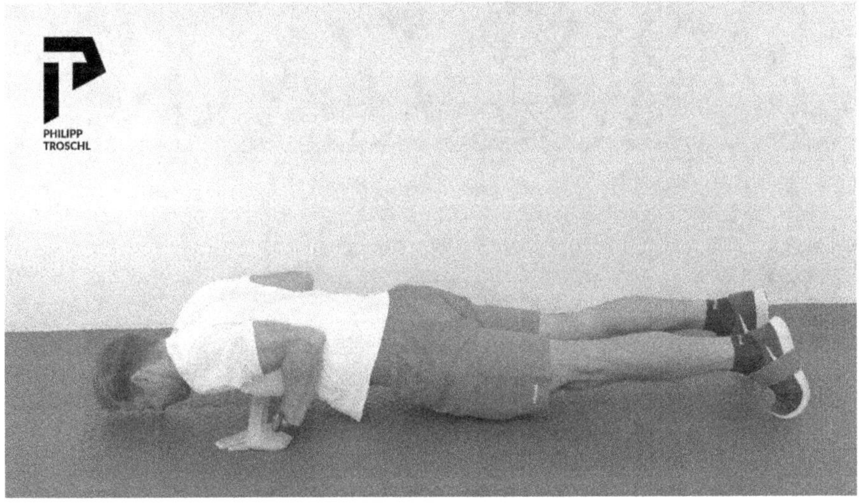

Clamshell (easy)

Starting position: Place the mini-band above your knees and lay down sideways. Bend your knees in a 90 degrees angle.

Exercise performance: Now lift your knees against the resistance of the mini-band and relax, but make sure that the knees do not touch if possible. Your feet should always touch each other. Repeat 15-20 times per side.

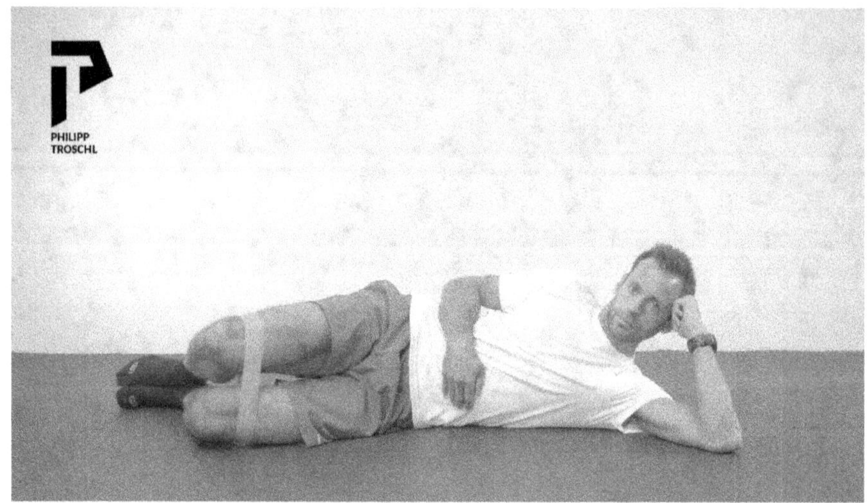

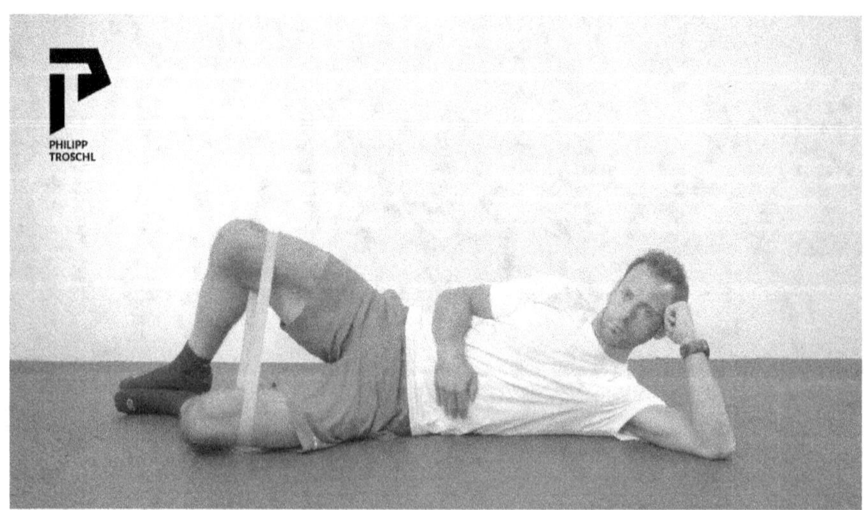

Leg lifts sideways (difficult)

Starting position: Place a mini-band above your knees and lay down sideways on the floor. Now lift your stretched legs.

Exercise performance: Now lift your stretched leg against the resistance of the mini-band and back together, but not fully. Repeat 10-15 times per side.

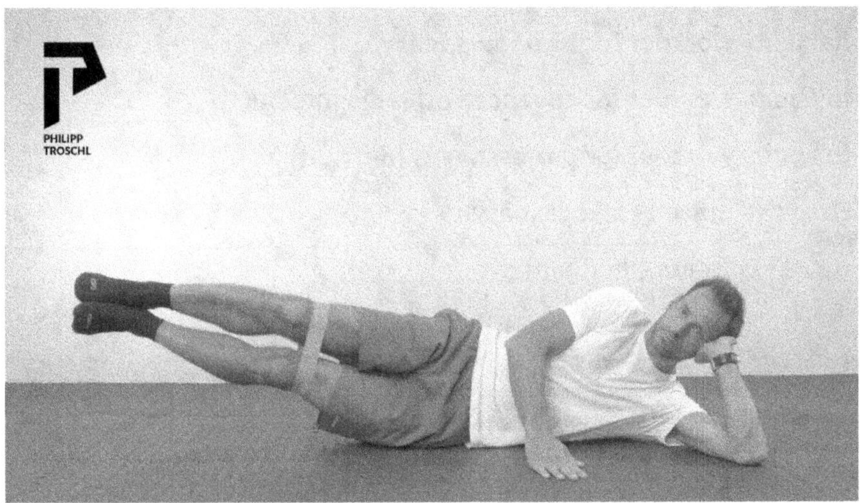

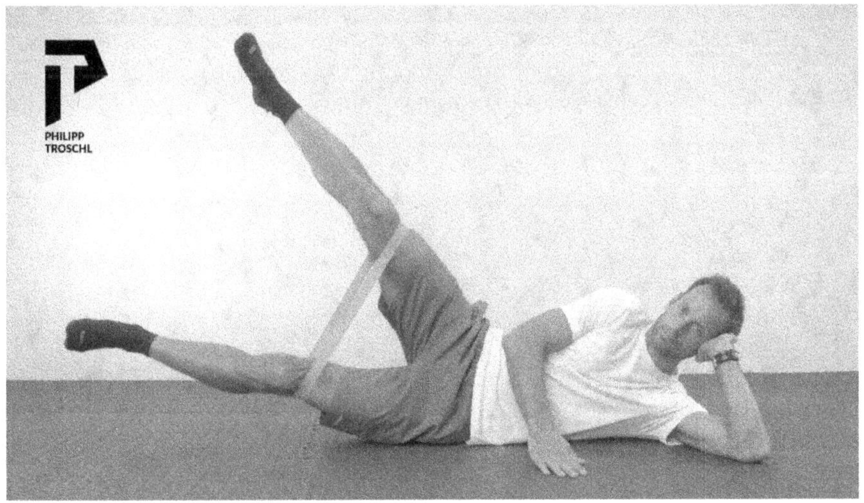

Mini-band Workout for at Home

In the following you will get six full body workouts in different levels of difficulty.

-5 min "anytime and anywhere" beginner workout (easy)

-full body workout for beginners (easy)

-full body workout for advanced athletes (medium)

-full body workout for professionals (difficult)

-Fit in the office Workout (easy)

-runner workout (medium)

Before every workout, it is recommended to warm up at least five minutes (see previous chapter). It not only prepares your body for training and reduces the risk of injury, but you will also improve your mobility. If you are short on time, you can also simply do 30 jumping jacks and/or start with a loose passage (low resistance of the band 20-30 repetitions).

5 min "anytime and anywhere" beginner workout with mini-band

Choose the strength of the mini-band so that 15-20 repetitions are possible for you to do. If you feel like you can do 30 repetitions easily, then choose a stronger band.

You perform 3 sets per exercise or do 3 runs of the entire exercise sequence!

Exercise performance:

15-20 repetitions per exercise

3 sets (runs)

	Leg lifts sideways – strengthening of the adductors
	Mini-band pulls
	Glute Bridge
	Russian Twist

Full Body Workout for Beginners

Choose the strength of the mini-band so that holding the exercise for 30 seconds or 15-20 repetitions are possible for you to do. If you feel like you can do 30 repetitions easily, or you can hold the exercise for 45 seconds or more, then choose a stronger band.

You perform 2 sets per exercise or do 2 runs of the entire exercise sequence!

Exercise performance:

2 runs: Version A or Version B, 1 min break in between. **Duration:** 16min (Version B)

Version A: 15-20 repetitions per exercise

Version B: HIIT: 30/15 (Training/Break)

	Monsterwalk
	Stars Excursion
	Leg lift sideways and strengthening of the adductors
	Mini-band pulls

	Squats
	Glute Bridge
	Quadruped arm pulls
	Arm pull in side plank position with bended knees
	Clamshell
	Russian Twist

Full Body Workout for Advanced Athletes

Exercise performance:

2 runs: Version A and Version B, 1 min break in between. **Duration:** 16min (Version B)

Version A: 15-20 repetitions per exercise

Version B: HIIT: 30/10 (Training/Break)

	Star Excursion
	Leg lift sideways and strengthening of the adductors
	Squat and shoulder strengthening
	Lunge and shoulder strengthening

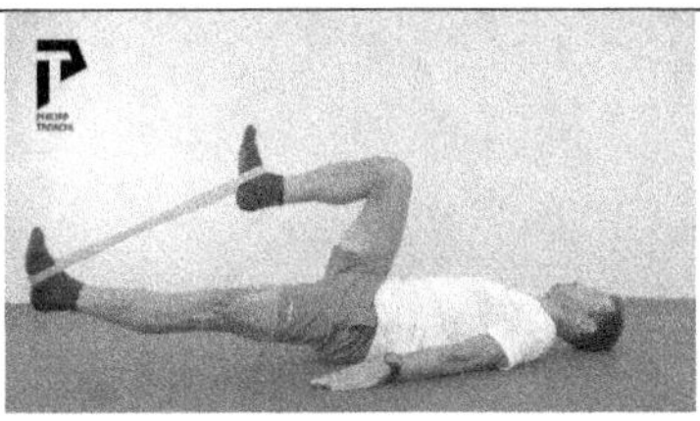	Leg stretching while lying down
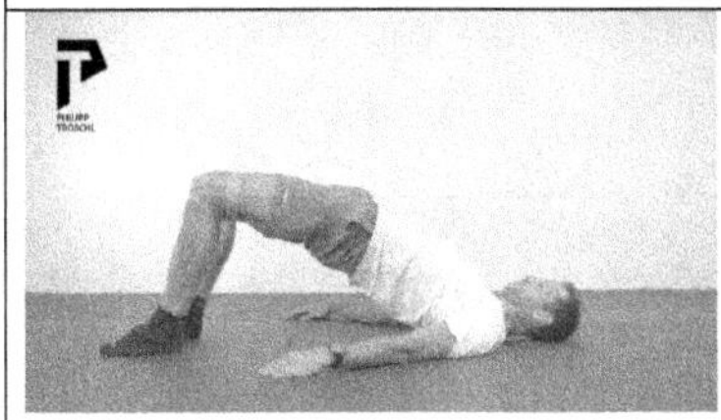	Glute Bridge
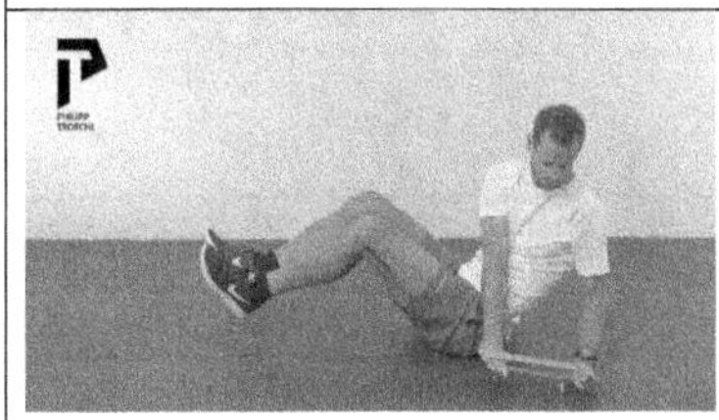	Russian Twist
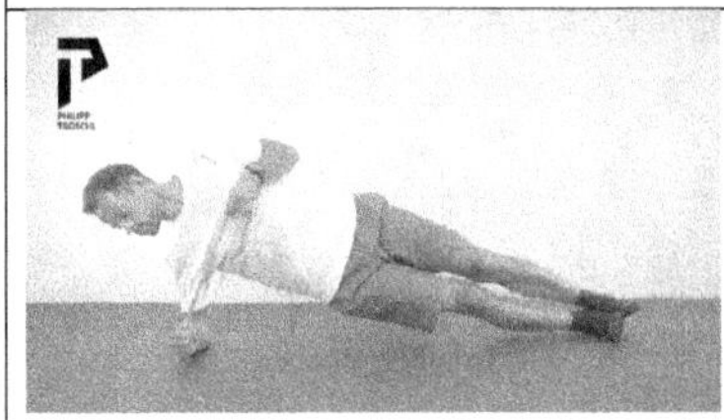	Arm pull in side push-up position and stretched legs
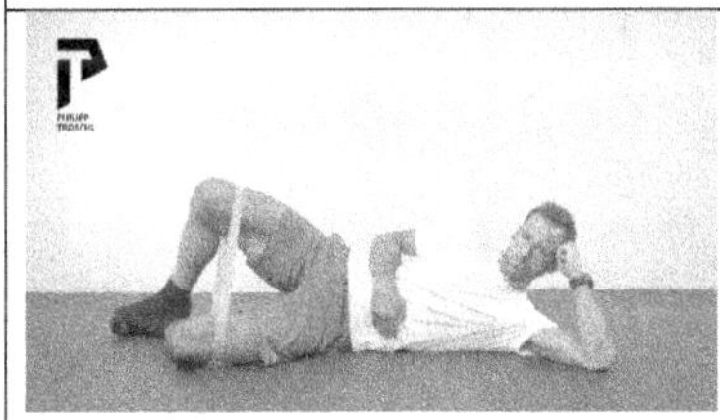	Knee lift
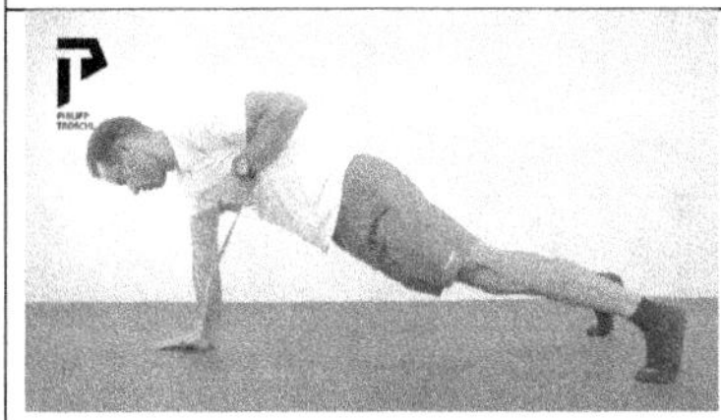	Arm pull in push-up position

Full Body Workout for Pros

Exercise performance:

2 runs: Version A and Version B, 1 min break in between. **Duration:** 16min (Version B)

Version A: 15-20 repetitions per exercise

Version B: HIIT: 30/10 (Training/Break)

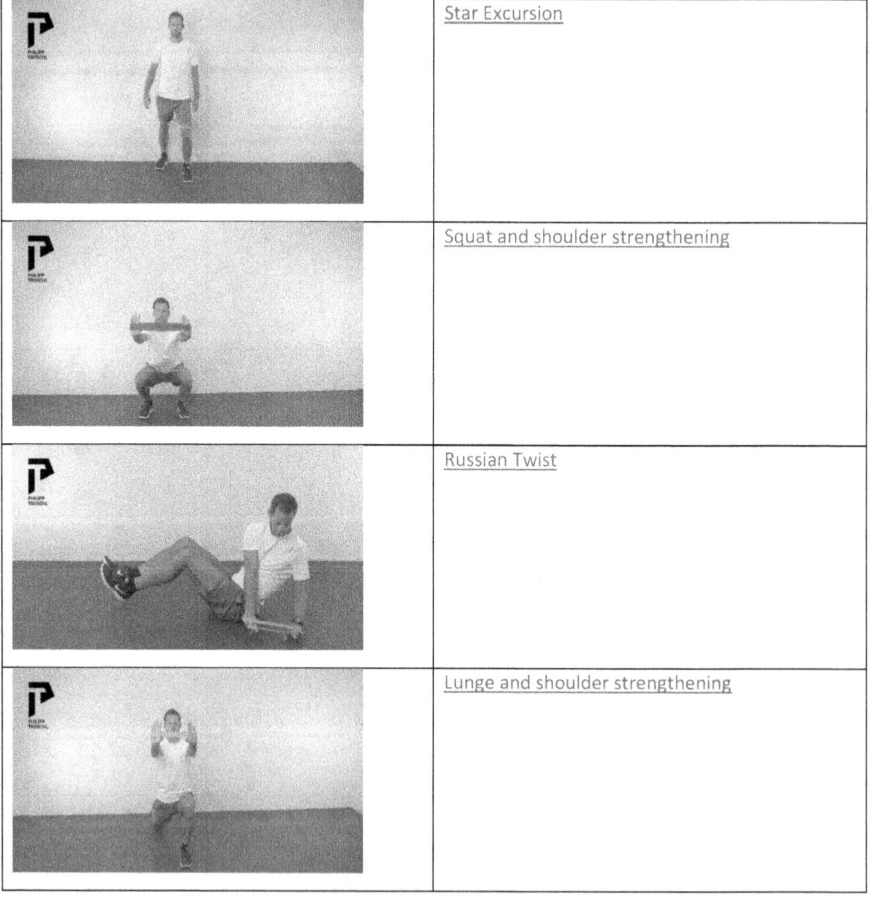

	Star Excursion
	Squat and shoulder strengthening
	Russian Twist
	Lunge and shoulder strengthening

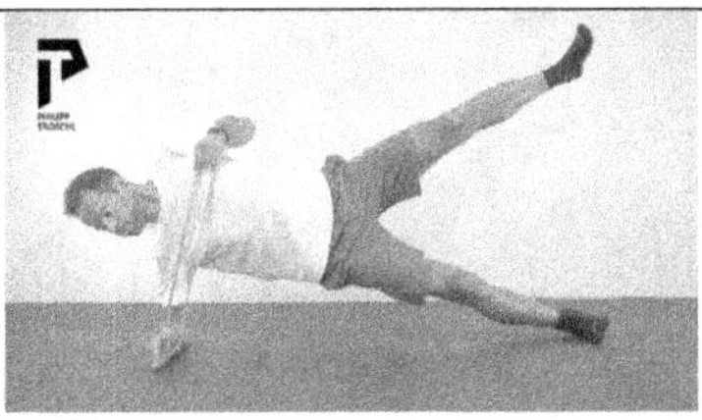	Leg lift in side plank position and arm pull Version B
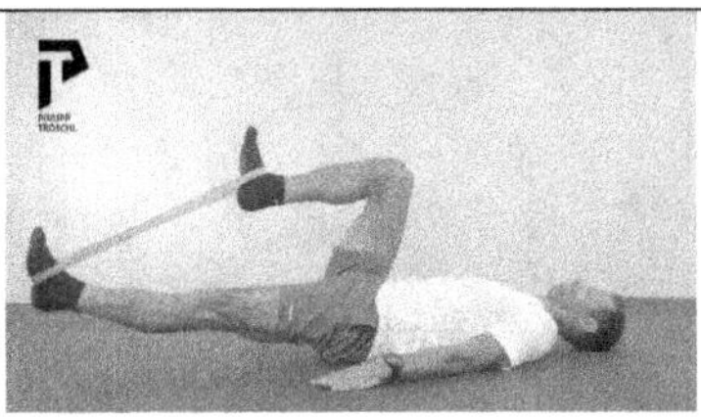	Leg stretch while lying down
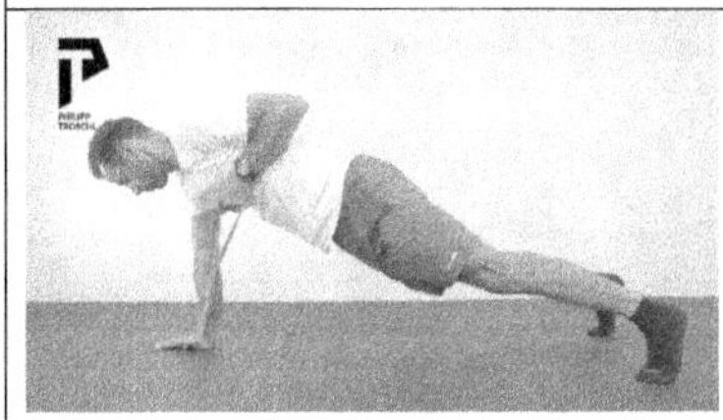	Push-up and arm pull right/left
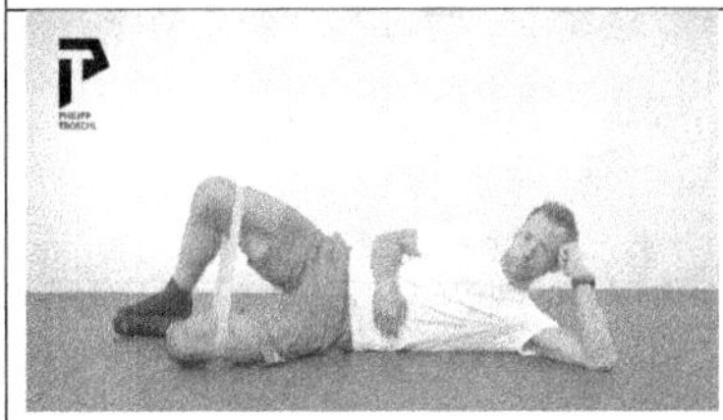	Clamshell
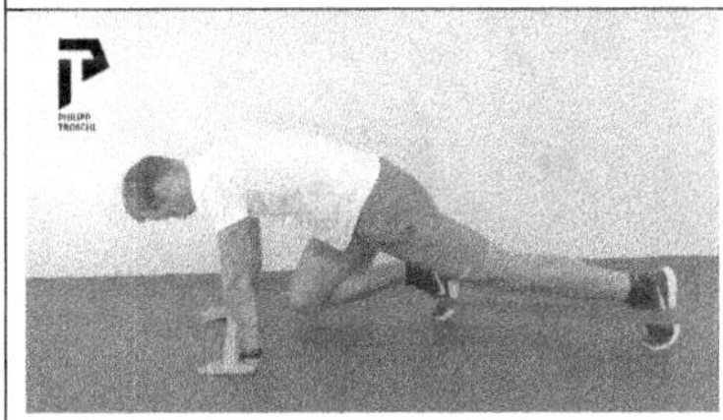	Pull-up knees alternately in plank position with push-up
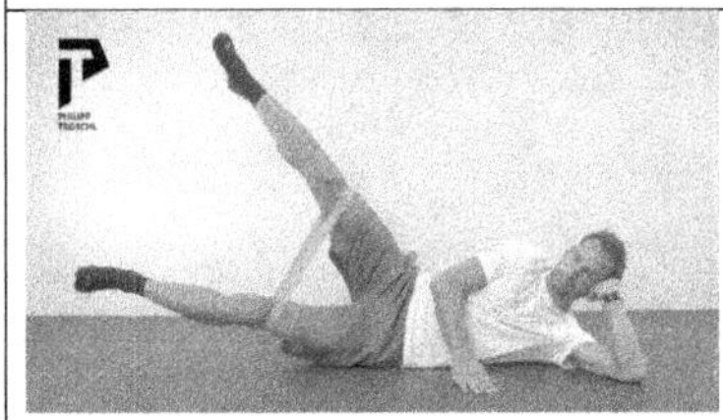	Leg lift sideways

Runner Mini-band Workout

Best if done before and after every running session.

Exercise performance:

2- 3 runs

15-20 repetitions per exercise

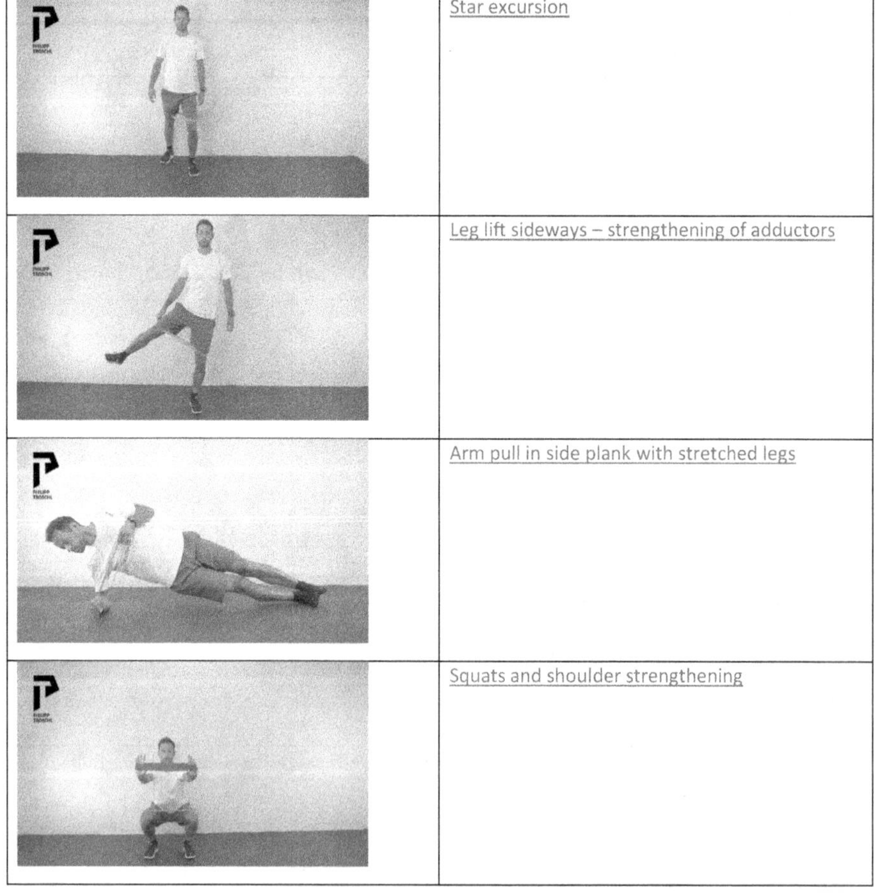

	Star excursion
	Leg lift sideways – strengthening of adductors
	Arm pull in side plank with stretched legs
	Squats and shoulder strengthening

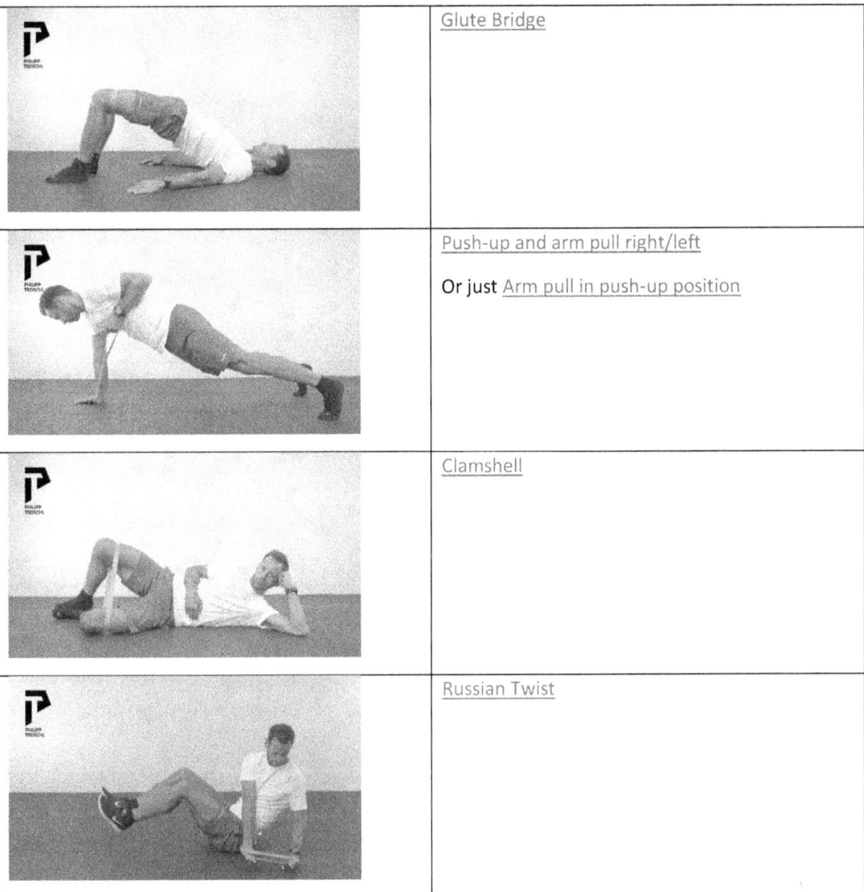

	Glute Bridge
	Push-up and arm pull right/left Or just Arm pull in push-up position
	Clamshell
	Russian Twist

Fit at Work Workout

Ideal for taking an active break from work for more energy.

<u>Exercise performance:</u>

2- 3 runs

15-20 repetitions per exercise

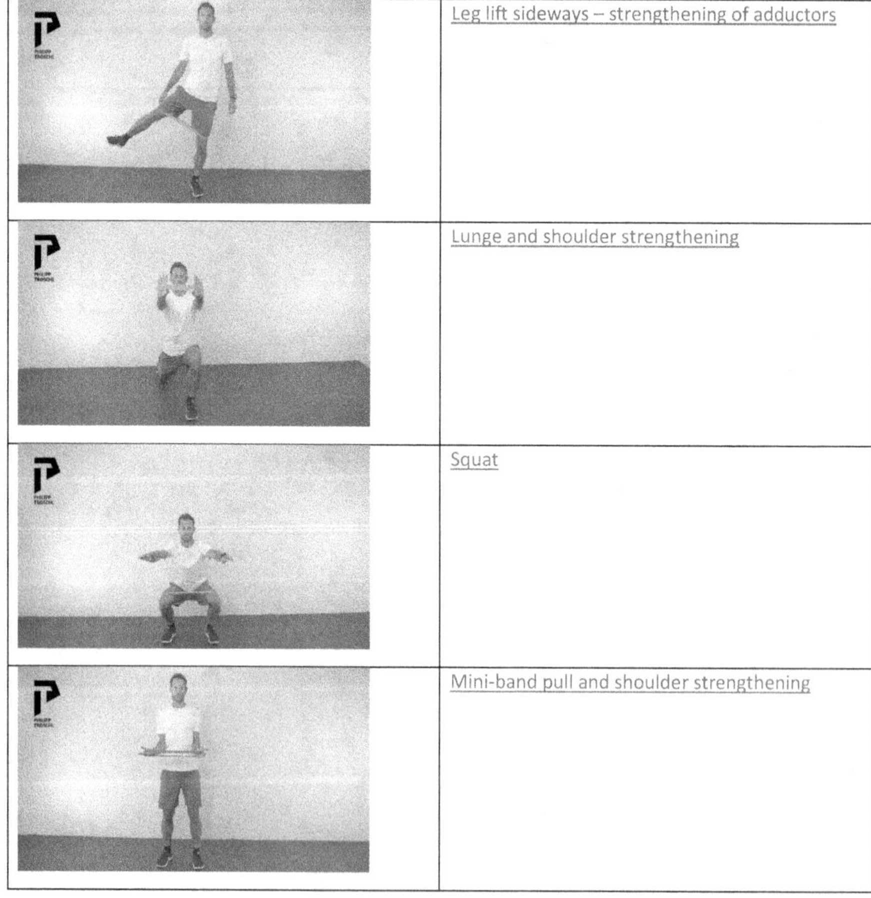

More information on this topic is available via my E-book: <u>E-Book: Fit im Büro</u>

This is how you motivate yourself for your set goals

At the end of this book I would like to motivate you a little and give you some tips on how to make your training successful with the right goals.

No matter what dreams and desires you have in your life, goals will help you achieve what you set out to do. In the specific case of fitness goals, they can be visions that will help you create a plan. This plan is then your guide that will take you step by step towards your vision of your dream body, your ideal weight or your athletic goal.

Even your training with the mini-band should pursue a goal!

I have successfully accompanied many people on their way to their goal and the first step was always the definition of the goal. The so-called **SMART method** has proven to be very useful in setting goals.

Setting Goals with the SMART method

If you simply set a goal and do nothing further, the probability that you will achieve it is extremely low. Goals must be clearly formulated, realistically achievable and have a fixed target date.

A very good method to implement and achieve a goal is to use the so-called **SMART method**.

Examples for a good and a bad formulated goal setting:

-Bad: I will lose weight

-Better: I will train 3 times a week (Mon, Wed, Fri at 6 PM) starting from 1. July for three months until the 1. October, in order to lose 6 kg.

Or

-Bad: I would like to eat more healthy

-Better: I will not eat any sugar, wheat, alcohol and processed and packaged food from this day on, for 30 days, in order to lose 2kg and feeling healthier.

This is why it is important that you achieve your goals

Whether you want to get fitter, lose weight, finish a sports competition, achieving your goal is very important for your self-confidence. If you reach it, you will be satisfied and happy. It will also fill you with pride.

If you pursue and achieve goals in one area, it is often easier to achieve goals in other areas too. No matter what goal and in which area you want to achieve it, the process is usually similar and always requires a certain consistency and regularity.

If you reach your fitness goal, you will not only become fitter, your posture and self-confidence will also change a lot!

Never give up!

If you don't achieve your goals, you lose self-confidence. This makes it more difficult to achieve further goals. It starts a downward spiral. In the worst case, you lose faith in yourself. It must not come so far. Therefore: "Never give up!

Achieving your goals will make you stronger!

People who set fitness goals on a regular basis usually have a good physical fitness level. They are motivated, brimming with self-confidence and regularly set themselves new, more demanding goals. This allows their personality to grow. People who regularly set themselves goals and achieve them are self-confident.

The biggest hurdle in the implementation of goals is a spongy, unclear formulation. This is immediately followed by inconsistency and excuses due to lack of time or other things. Therefore, your goal must have a certain importance for you. If it is really important to you, you should be prepared to take the necessary consistency for it. When you are struggling to apply the consistency, the goal is probably not important enough for you.

"If you do not give your goal the necessary priority, then you will probably give up soon."

That is why you should always remember:

"Formulate your goals clearly, make a plan and stick to it. Then you will achieve your goals!"

Not only will you feel healthier and more fit, but also this will influence other parts of your life positively too.

If it is a fitness goal that you have achieved, you will feel fitter, healthier, slimmer, in short, simply more vital! But, no matter what kind of goal you achieve, there are many benefits to not only setting goals, but also achieving them:

9 Reasons why it is important to set your training goals!

Your overall fitness improves

Your health awareness improves

You are going to feel more vital

You are going to be proud of yourself

It encourages you in your actions

Further goals are going to be easier for you in the future

Faith in yourself increases

Your self-confidence is going to be strengthened

It will also have a positive effect on many other areas of your life!

Have fun implementing the exercises and tips from this book!

What is next?

Step 1:

Subscribe to my newsletter on my homepage to receive regular updates and tips on fitness and health.

Step 2:

Send me an email (info@philipp-troschl.at) and you will receive a free 4-week plan to help you implement the content.

Step 3:

Start your journey on your way to more energy at work and everyday life.

About the Author

I, Philipp Troschl have dedicated my life to exercise and health. As a sports scientist, personal coach, life coach and state-certified trainer, I have been working with private individuals and companies for many years. My work focuses on workplace health promotion, functional training, stabilization training, holistic training and various aspects of health.

In cooperation with insurance companies and educational institutions (University Sports Institute Klagenfurt) I offer courses and lectures on topics such as back fitness, fascial training, stabilization training and more.

References:

Fit mit dem Miniband, Marcel Doll

Optimales Training, Jürgen Weineck

Functional Training, Michael Boyle

Core Performance, Mark Verstegen

Links:

https://www.faz.net/aktuell/gesellschaft/gesundheit/nach-einer-dkv-studie-bewegen-sich-deutsche-kaum-14377616.html

I can recommend these mini-bands:

Griffin Minibands

For more information on this topic, I recommend this book: Fit mit dem Miniband (german only)

Photos:

Dieter Frank, Frank Film und Foto

Translation:
from German Naomi Köfler

 You can find more information about my work and tips for your fitness, well-being and health on:

Homepage: www.philipp-troschl.at

Facebook: https://www.facebook.com/progresstraining/

Instagram: https://www.instagram.com/philipp_troschl/

More books from the author Philipp Troschl:

-Fit at Work

Imprint

Published by:

Philipp Troschl

Evaweg 3

9020 Klagenfurt

info@philipp-troschl.at

www.ingramcontent.com/pod-product-compliance
Lightning Source LLC
Chambersburg PA
CBHW061735250726
48657CB00002B/941